CLINICAL MANAGEMENT OF ELECTROLYTE DISORDERS

DEVELOPMENTS IN CRITICAL CARE MEDICINE AND ANESTHESIOLOGY

Other volumes in this series:

Prakash, Omar (ed.): Applied Physiology in Clinical Respiratory Care. 1982.
ISBN 90–247–2662–X.

McGeown, Mary G.: Clinical Management of Electrolyte Disorders. 1983.
ISBN 0–89838–559–8.

Klain, Miroslav: High Frequency Ventilation.

Scheck, P.A., Sjöstrand, U.H., and Smith, R.B. (eds.): Perspectives in High Frequency Ventilation. 1983. ISBN 0–89838–571–7.

Stanley, Th.H. and Petty, W.C. (eds.): New Anesthetic Agents, Devices and Monitoring Techniques. 1983. ISBN 0–89838–566–0.

CLINICAL MANAGEMENT OF ELECTROLYTE DISORDERS

by

MARY G. McGEOWN, MD, PhD, FRCP, FRCP Ed, FRCPI

Renal Unit, Belfast City Hospital
Belfast

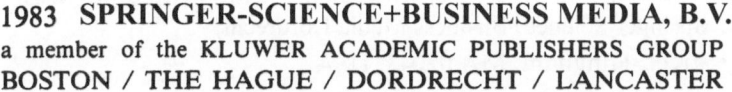1983 **SPRINGER-SCIENCE+BUSINESS MEDIA, B.V.**
a member of the KLUWER ACADEMIC PUBLISHERS GROUP
BOSTON / THE HAGUE / DORDRECHT / LANCASTER

Distributors

for the United States and Canada: Kluwer Boston, Inc., 190 Old Derby Street, Hingham, MA 02043, USA
for all other countries: Kluwer Academic Publishers Group, Distribution Center, P.O.Box 322, 3300 AH Dordrecht, The Netherlands

Library of Congress Cataloging in Publication Data

```
McGeown, Mary G.
   Clinical management of electrolyte disorders.

   (Developments in critical care medicine and
anesthesiology)
   Bibliography: p.
   1. Water-electrolyte imbalances--Treatment.
2. Electrolyte therapy.  3. Intravenous therapy.
I. Title.  II. Series.  [DNLM: 1. Water-electrolyte
imbalance--Therapy.  WD 220 M478c]
RC630.M4  1983      616      82-19012
```

ISBN 978-94-009-6701-4   ISBN 978-94-009-6699-4 (eBook)
DOI 10.1007/978-94-009-6699-4

Copyright

To my husband, Max Freeland

Preface

Serious disturbances of fluid and electrolyte balance are frequently encountered in acutely ill patients; somewhat less often in the chronically sick. There seems to be a trend for such cases to increase, due probably to an increase in major surgical procedures on older patients whose renal function is less than adequate.

There are already many publications dealing with the physiology of the homeostasis of fluid and electrolytes, and others dealing with the clinical aspects of the subject. It is often assumed that a knowledge of the basic principles of physiology will enable the doctor to prescribe suitable intravenous therapy. In practice this is often found not to be so and the evidence for this is the frequency of calls for help with electrolyte problems from well-qualified and experienced doctors who are undoubtedly equipped with adequate or even excellent knowledge of the basic principles involved. It is not an unusual observation that knowledge of theory and principles does not necessarily lead to successful practice in this or any other art or craft.

Most doctors already possess knowledge of the physiology of the internal environment, but some are aware of being unable to deal effectively with clinical problems related to fluid and electrolyte disturbances and seek guidance to translate theoretical knowledge into practice.

This book is offered, not without diffidence, to those who experience the need for a simple manual on intravenous therapy, emphasizing the clinical aspects of the work rather than the basic physiology and biochemistry. For deeper study many excellent texts are available, a useful selection of which is given in the accompanying bibliography.

Belfast   Mary G. McGeown
June 1982

Acknowledgements

I am happy to acknowledge the generous help of friends and colleagues. Dr C.C. Doherty read the second draft and made many useful suggestions. Dr D. Neill's comments on Chapters 1 and 7 were helpful and Mr S. Nesbitt gave invaluable detailed help with these chapters.

I am grateful to Doctors E. Whitehead, C. Farnan and P. Freeland for their help with correction of the final text.

I wish to thank Mrs Sylvia Crowe for her patience and for her careful typing of the text.

Write the vision, and make it plain upon tables,
that he may run that readeth it

Habakkuk ii, 2

Table of contents

1. Basic information relating to body fluids

Body fluids are solutions where the solvent is water in which particles (solutes) are dissolved.

1. Volume

In physiological terms this means the volume of water and its dissolved solutes in the body as a whole, or in a compartment of the body. It is measured in litres (1) or millilitres (ml).

2. Solutes

These are molecules or fragments of molecules. When molecules dissolve in water they dissociate to a greater or lesser extent into their component parts. They then become electrically charged and are known as ions. The ion may be a single atom, e.g., sodium (Na, carrying a positive charge), or may be a combination of atoms, e.g., the hydroxyl ion (OH^-, carrying a negative charge). An ion carrying a positive electrical charge is called a *cation*. An ion carrying a negative electrical charge is called an *anion*.

3. Mole

The unit of mass is the mole, or the molecular weight expressed in grams. For example, one mole of sodium chloride is contained in 58.5 grams, i.e., the sum of the atomic weights of sodium (23) and chloride (35.5). In the case of ions one mole is the atomic weight expressed in grams.

Many substances are present in biological fluids in amounts very much smaller than the mole. The smaller units of mass are each subdivisions by 1000 of the one above.

1 mole	(mol)	=	1000 millimoles	(mmol)
1 millimole	$(10^{-3}\,mol)$	=	1000 micromoles	(μmol)
1 micromole	$(10^{-6}\,mol)$	=	1000 nanomoles	(nmol)

$$1 \text{ nanomole} \quad (10^{-9} \text{ mol}) \quad = \quad 1000 \text{ picomoles} \quad (\text{pmol})$$
$$1 \text{ picomole} \quad (10^{-12} \text{ mol})$$

4. Solution

The concentrations of solutes in biological solutions are expressed in moles, or fractions of a mole, per litre (mol/l). The solutions of electrolytes with which we will be concerned are present in concentrations of millimoles per litre (mmol/l). Where the exact chemical structure of a biological substance is unknown the concentration is expressed as grams (or its subdivisions) per litre.

This system of expressing concentrations of solutes in biological fluids in terms of molar concentration, the Système Internationale d'Unités (SI), has superseded the older system where the concentration was expressed in grams (or milligrams) per 100 ml, or mEq/l.

5. Equivalent

Early chemists more than 200 years ago discovered that the weights of two elements which combine chemically with each other are always in a fixed ratio. For example 1 g of hydrogen combines with 35.5 g of chlorine to form hydrochloric acid. It was later discovered that the amounts which combine are in fact the atomic weights or some ratio of the atomic weights of the elements. This concept of combining or equivalent weight continues to be used.

The equivalent (Eq) is the mass of an anion which combines with 1 g of hydrogen (H^+) or that of a cation which combines with 17 g of hydroxyl (OH^-).

The equivalent therefore is a mass defined in terms in the amount of electrical charge carried, and one equivalent equals one Faraday (96500 coulombs). It assumes that electrolytes dissociate completely in solution, which is not strictly true. Nevertheless, the terms equivalent and milliequivalent are useful in the study of the transport of electrolytes across membranes.

The weight of a salt in milligrams can be converted into milliequivalents by dividing by molecular weight and multiplying by the valency.

For example:

$$Na\,Cl = Na \text{ (atomic weight 23, valency 1)}$$
$$+ \, Cl \text{ (atomic weight 35.5, valency 1)}$$
$$= 58.5$$

$$\frac{1000}{58.5} \times 1 = 17.1 \text{ mEq}$$

$$1000 \text{ mg NaCl} = 17.1 \text{ mEq}$$

6. Osmosis

This term is used to describe the spontaneous flow of a solvent into a solution, or from a more dilute into a more concentrated solution, when the two liquids are separated from each other by a suitable membrane. Strictly speaking, osmosis refers to the flow of solvent only. If solute also moves, in the opposite direction, this is referred to as diffusion. A membrane which permits osmosis to occur, that is free passage of the solvent, e.g., water, but not the dissolved substance, e.g., sugar, is said to be semipermeable.

7. Osmotic pressure

This is defined as the excess pressure which must be applied to a solution to prevent the passage into it of solvent when it is separated from the solvent by a perfectly semipermeable membrane. Plant and animal cells are enclosed in membranes which are largely but not completely semipermeable. In a normal cell the pressure of the cell water is such that the cell constituents are pressed against the membrane, producing the normal turgidity of cells. If the normal cell is then placed in water or in a solution of osmotic pressure less than that exerted by the solution in the cell, there will be a tendency for water to enter leading to increased pressure within the cell (cellular overhydration). If on the other hand the cell is placed in a solution having a higher osmotic pressure, water will pass through the cell membrane into the solution, causing the cell to shrink and become dehydrated (cellular underhydration). When diffusion takes place across the cell membrane until there is a uniform mixture on both sides of the membrane then a state of osmotic equilibirium is reached.

8. Osmolarity, osmolality

Osmolarity is a measurement of the osmotic activity of a solution and is determined by the number of molecules or ions of solute present per unit volume of solution. One mole of a substance which dissociates almost completely, such as sodium chloride into sodium and chloride, contains 2 osmoles. One mole of a substance which does not dissociate, such as glucose, contains one osmole.

The addition of a solute to a liquid solvent reduces the freezing point of the solution below that of the pure solvent, the reduction being proportional to the concentration of the solute. This relationship holds true for a single solute or for a mixture of solutes. The measurement of the change in freezing point can thus be used for the estimation of the concentration of ions and molecules in solution. An *osmolar solution* contains *one osmole dissolved in water and made up to one litre.*

8.1. Osmolarity

Osmolarity, therefore, is the term used to describe the concentration of active particles in *one litre of solution*. An osmolar solution contains one osmole dissolved in water and made up to one litre.

It has been recommended that the expression of osmolarity and osmolality in terms of osmoles be discontinued and the term mole used instead.

8.2. Osmolality

Osmolality is the term used to describe the concentration of active particles in *one kilogram of solvent*. For simple solutions the difference between osmolarity and osmolality is so small that it can be neglected. In complicated biological solutions containing many solutes, such as plasma, the difference is considerable and the more correct measurement is that expressed per kilogram of solvent, i.e., *osmolality*.

9. Isotonicity, hypertonicity, hypotonicity

In normal circumstances the fluids within the different fluid compartments are in osmotic equilibrium with each other and in this state of normal balance the fluids are said to be *isotonic* with respect to each other. If, however, the normal balance is disturbed and there is an excess of solute over the normal concentration in one compartment, then the fluid in that compartment is said to be *hypertonic* with respect to normal and initially with respect to the other compartments. Similarly a loss of solute from a fluid compartment renders the fluid *hypotonic* with respect to normal. The osmolality of body fluids varies between 280 and 300 mmol/kg H_2O. Females have values 5 to 10 mmol/kg H_2O below that of males.

An increase in osmolality in any one fluid compartment immediately leads to withdrawal of water from the adjacent compartment. The solute, causing the change in osmolality, if freely diffusible, will diffuse out of the compartment and eventually equilibrium concentrations on each side of the membrane will be restored. However, as water diffuses at twice the rate of ions the immediate effect is usually a change in intracellular hydration. Likewise a reduction in osmolality in one compartment will be followed by loss of fluid to the adjacent (relatively hypertonic) compartment.

10. Oncotic pressure

The osmotic activity of the fluid in the body compartments is however, more complicated than the above description would suggest, because of the presence of molecules such as proteins which are too large to pass through the cell membranes dividing intracellular from extracellular fluid, and extracellular fluid from the vascular compartment. These exert a small osmotic effect as particles, which

Table 1. Average composition of plasma.

	mEq/l	mmol/l
Cations		
Na	140	140
K	4	4
Ca	10^a	2.5
Mg	1.6	0.8
Anions		
Cl	103	103
HCO_3	26	26
PO_4	4^a	1.5
SO_4	1	0.5
Protein	16	16
Organic acids		3

^{a} mg/100 ml.

contributes to movement of water into their compartment. This small net osmotic effect due to proteins is referred to as the *colloid osmotic pressure* or *oncotic pressure*.

11. Cell membrane pumps

The cell membrane does not behave simply as an inert semipermeable membrane through which water and ions diffuse passively until equilibrium is reached. There are cell membrane pumps which regulate the concentrations of certain ions, particularly sodium and potassium, and calcium and magnesium, so that the ionic composition of intracellular fluid is quite different to that of extracellular fluid (Tables 1 and 2). The regulation of these pumps is still poorly understood but it is probable that aldosterone regulates the sodium/potassium pump, and parathyroid hormone the calcium/magnesium pump. Pumps regulating movements of anions also exist.

12. Role of enzymes

The metabolic activity within cells is under the control of enzymes. A consideration of enzyme activity is outside the scope of this book, but it should be remembered that enzyme systems are very sensitive to alterations of pH.

13. Acid/base

The definitions used here are the chemical ones proposed by Brønsted in 1928. An *acid* is a hydrogen ion (proton) donor, i.e., it is a molecule which can give off a

Table 2. Average composition of intracellular fluid of a muscle cell.

	mEq/kg cell water	mmol/l cell water
Cations		
Na	32	10
K	102	160
Ca	2	
Mg	28	
Anions		
Cl	$\pm$ 0–3	$\pm$ 0–3
HCO_3	10	10
PO_4	105	
SO_4	20	
Protein	65	

Note: Different values are given by different authors, probably because age and sex, which have recently been shown to be of consequence, have not been taken into account.

hydrogen ion. A *base* is a hydrogen ion (proton) acceptor, i.e., it can take up a hydrogen ion.
Example:

Acid		H^+ + Base
H_2CO_3	$\rightleftharpoons$	$H^+ + HCO_3^-$
H_3PO_4	$\rightleftharpoons$	$H^+ + H_2PO_4$
(Hydrogen ion donors)		(Hydrogen ion acceptors)

In both equations the anion left after the loss of hydrogen ion is by definition a base as it will accept a hydrogen ion when the reaction is reversed.

An acid, such as HCl, in an aqueous solution dissociates into its component ions, in this case H^+ and Cl^-. The strength of an acid depends on how completely it dissociates and the concentration of hydrogen ions it liberates in solution.

A Danish biochemist, Sorensen, noted in 1909 that minute changes in hydrogen ion concentration affected activities of enzymes, changes of the order of 0.01 (10^{-2}) to 0.0000001 (10^{-7}) mole per litre being important. He called the -2 and -7 the hydrogen power (in his French text, 'puissance Hydrogen') which he shortened to the term pH, dropping the minus sign.

pH is defined as the negative logarithm of the hydrogen ion concentration in moles per litre of solution.

A strong acid such as 0.1 molar HCL has a pH of 1. A strong base such as 0.1 molar NaOH has a pH of 13.

The physiological range of pH is narrow and lies between 7.38 and 7.42, equivalent to a hydrogen ion concentration of 42 to 38 nanomoles per litre (the solid part of the pH line in Fig. 1) Under disease conditions the pH may vary between 6.9 and 7.6.

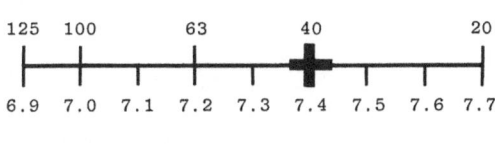

Fig. 1. The pH range in body fluids. The physiological range (7.38–7.42) is shown by the thick line.

13.1. Acidosis

An increase in the concentration of hydrogen ions in plasma is known as *acidosis*. This abnormally high concentration of hydrogen ions is denoted by a *low* pH value, i.e., a shift to the left in the pH range shown in Fig. 1.

13.2. Alkalosis

A decrease in the concentration of hydrogen ions in plasma is known as *alkalosis*. This abnormally low concentration of hydrogen ions is denoted by a *high* pH value, i.e., a shift to the right in the pH range shown in Fig. 1.

13.3. Buffers

The presence of a buffer in a solution decreases the pH change which tends to be produced by addition of either an acid or a base. A buffer is a compound which dissociates only partially in solution. It is a mixture of a weak acid and its alkali salt or of a weak base and its acid salt. The important buffers in the body fluids are mixtures of weak acids and their alkali salts – carbonic acid and sodium (or potassium) bicarbonate, mono-hydrogen phosphate and dihydrogen phosphate, proteins and their sodium or potassium salts, haemoglobin and its salts.

The continuous metabolic processes within cells results in production of H^+ ion which must be neutralised by the buffer systems. The bicarbonate/carbonic acid buffer system is the most important one in extracellular fluid. The reaction set up leads to the production of water and carbon dioxide, which is excreted by the lungs. Examples:

$$HCL + NaHCO_3 \rightarrow H_2CO_3 + NaCl \qquad H_2CO_3 \rightarrow H_2O + CO_2$$
$$NaOH + H_2CO_3 \rightarrow NaHCO_3 + H_2O$$

The bicarbonate ion plays a very important part in the maintenance of plasma pH close to 7.4.

The phosphate buffer system is especially important in the excretion of hydrogen ion by the renal tubules.

13.4. Anion gap

The cations and anions in plasma are present in electrical equivalence, the average values being shown in Table 1. The sum of the cations in millimoles per litre equals the sum of anions. The actual sums may be more than that shown in the table, when water has been lost by dehydration, or less when excess of water has been given.

Anions such as phosphates, sulphates, organic acids and proteins are not usually measured as part of an 'electrolyte block' in clinical laboratories. The sum of the measured cations, Na^+, K^+ and Ca^+, in normal circumstances is greater than the sum of the measured anions, HCO_3^- and Cl^- by about 16 mmol/l or less – the *normal anion gap*.

$$Na^+ + K^+ + Ca^{++} = 140 + 3.5 + 2.5 \text{ mmol/l}$$
$$= 146 \text{ mmol/l}$$

$$HCO_3^- + Cl^- = 25 + 105 \text{ mmol/l}$$
$$= 130 \text{ mmol/l}$$

$$(Na^+ + K^+ + Ca^{++}) - (HCO_3^- + Cl^-) = 146\text{–}130 \text{ mmol/l}$$
$$= 16 \text{ mmol/l}$$

An anion gap of less than 9 mmol/l is very unlikely and is probably due to laboratory error.

When HCO_3^- falls there is often a compensatory rise in Cl^- (*hyperchloraemic acidosis*) and the anion gap remains normal. A compensatory rise in chloride occurs when acidosis is due to renal or gastrointestinal loss of bicarbonate (e.g., renal tubular acidosis, diarrhoea or fistula loss), or to administration of chloride.

Increased anion gap.
An increase in the anion gap is usually due to an increase in unmeasured anions, such as aceto-acetate in diabetic ketoacidosis; phosphate, sulphate and organic acids in renal failure; ketoglutaric acid in hepatic failure.

An increased anion gap may be due to ingestion of drugs such as salicylates leading to keto-acid production, or methanol, leading to formic acid production. Penicillin and carbenicillin also appear as unmeasured anions.

13.5. Regulation of acid/base

The most important buffer system in extracellular fluid is H_2CO_3/HCO_3^-. The factors which determine whether a buffer pair will release or bind H^+ depends on the dissociation constant (K) for that pair and the H^+ concentration in the solutions. For the carbonic acid/bicarbonate buffer pair the formula is:

$$H_2CO_3 \underset{k2}{\overset{k1}{\rightleftharpoons}} H^+ + HCO_3^-$$

Henderson modified this to:

$$(H^+) = K\frac{[H_2CO_3]}{[HCO_3^-]} \qquad K = \frac{k1}{k2}$$

Hasselbalch modified this to the negative logarithm form:

$$pH = pK + \log\frac{[HCO_3^-]}{[H_2CO_3]} \quad \text{where } p = -\log$$

The constant pK is dependent on pH, temperature and ionic strength in solution. In plasma at 37°C, pK^1, as pK is known when conditions are defined, is 6.1. H_2CO_3 is in equilibrium with the CO_2 in solution which in turn depends on P_{CO_2}. Therefore

$$H_2CO_3 = S.P_{CO_2} \quad S = \text{solubility coefficient for } CO_2 \text{ at } 37°C$$

The Henderson-Hasselbalch equation can now be modified to:

$$pH = pK^1 + \log\frac{[HCO_3^-]}{S.P_{CO_2}}$$

The variables $[HCO_3^-]$ and P_{CO_2} are regulated by the kidneys and lungs respectively, to maintain the blood pH at about 7.4. Changes in pH are defended rapidly by the buffers in blood but more slowly by respiratory regulation and by renal regulation.

13.5.1. Regulation of acid/base by the kidneys

Hydrogen ion is present in the diet and is produced by metabolism of food and body tissues. A normal individual consuming a normal diet has to excrete about 60 mmol of hydrogen ion daily to remain in balance. A high protein diet increases the amount of hydrogen ion produced. The excess hydrogen ion has to be excreted by the kidneys.

The glomerular filtrate in the proximal renal tubule contains sodium ions and bicarbonate ions at the concentrations present in extracellular fluid (140 and 25 mmol/l respectively). The sodium concentration in the cells lining the renal tubules (Fig. 2) is much lower (10 mmol/l), therefore sodium diffuses into the tubule cells and is removed into the renal extracellular (peritubular) fluid by the cell membrane pump, which maintains intracellular sodium level. Within the tubule cell carbon dioxide (CO_2) is combined with water (H_2O) under the action of carbonic anhydrase to form carbonic acid (H_2CO_3). The H_2CO_3 thus produced dissociates into bicarbonate ions (HCO_3^-) and hydrogen ions (H^+), the latter diffusing into the

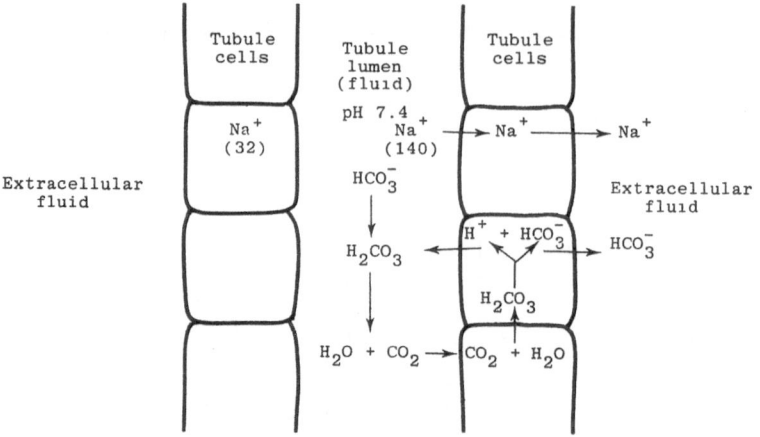

Fig. 2. Conservation of bicarbonate in proximal renal tubules.

lumen of the tubule in exchange for sodium ions

$$CO_2 + H_2O \rightleftharpoons H_2CO_3 \rightleftharpoons H^+ + HCO_3{}^-$$

This exchange of sodium for hydrogen ion and reabsorption of bicarbonate throughout the tubules conserves essential bicarbonate buffer.

Excess hydrogen ion is excreted throughout the tubules in 3 ways.

13.5.1.1. Excretion of hydrogen ion as ammonium. Ammonia is produced within tubule cells by the action of the enzymes glutaminase and deaminase on glutamine and amino acids respectively. The ammonia diffuses into tubular fluid where it combines with free hydrogen ions (produced initially within tubule cells by the action of carbonic anhydrase on H_2CO_3 as above) and is excreted as ammonium ion (Fig. 3).

13.5.1.2. Excretion of titratable acid. Hydrogen ion is excreted into the distal tubules and combined with conjugate bases to form conjugate acids. These acids form the titratable acid in urine.

(An acid dissociates into H^+ plus base, the action being reversible:

$$Acid \rightleftharpoons H^+ + base$$

The anion left after dissociation of hydrogen ion is by definition a base, being an acceptor of hydrogen ion. The acid and its base are known as conjugate acid and conjugate base, respectively.

The most important of the conjugate acid/base systems in urine is the monobasic/dibasic phosphate buffer system

$$H^+ + PO_4{}^{--} \rightleftharpoons H_2PO_4{}^-$$

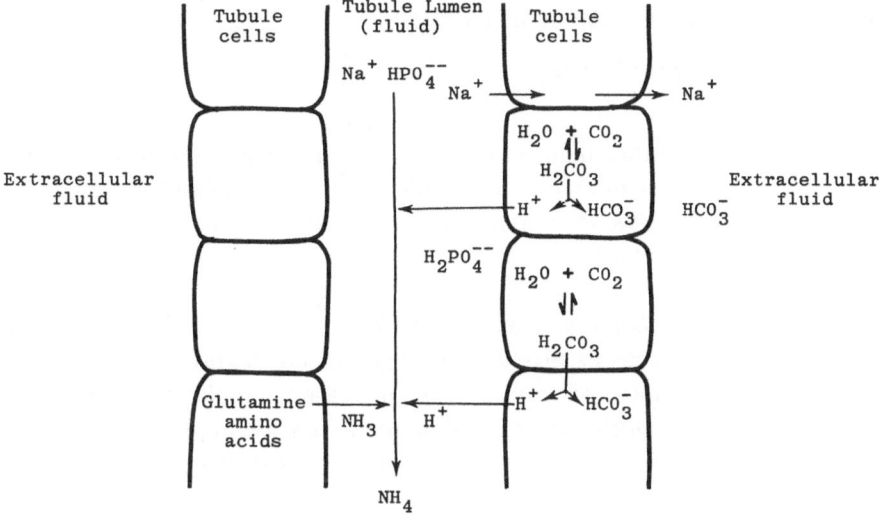

Fig. 3. Excretion of hydrogen ion in distal renal tubules.

As in the proximal tubule cells, hydrogen ion is generated within distal tubule cells by the action of carbonic anhydrase on CO_2 and H_2O, and excreted into the tubule lumen where it combines with monobasic HPO_4 to form dibasic H_2PO_4 which is then excreted (Fig. 3). The bicarbonate diffuses into extracellular fluid.

13.5.1.3. Free hydrogen ion. A very small amount of free hydrogen ion is excreted in the urine. Even when urine is excreted at maximum acidity (pH 4.0) only 0.1 mmol/l H^+ is excreted in this way.

13.5.2. Regulation of acid/base by the lungs
In the Henderson-Hasselbalch equation P_{CO_2} is regulated by the lungs. Respiratory acidosis and respiratory alkalosis are due to changes in excretion of CO_2 by the lungs. CO_2 when in solution is in equilibrium with carbonic acid, H_2CO_3.

13.5.2.1. Respiratory acidosis. Respiratory acidosis occurs when CO_2 tension (P_{CO_2}) is increased and pH falls. This is the result of failure of the lungs to excrete metabolically produced CO_2. Production of CO_2 is fairly constant and respiratory acidosis usually is the result of defective ventilation.

When CO_2 excretion is less than CO_2 production, P_{CO_2} increases – *hypercapnia*. When hypercapnia becomes steady, CO_2 excretion equals production at a new equilibrium because the P_{CO_2} carried to the lung vascular bed has increased sufficiently to allow excretion to equal production despite decreased alveolar ventilation.

The increase in P_{CO_2} leads to an increase in dissolved CO_2 and shifts the equilibrium towards production of H_2CO_3:

$$CO_2 + H_2O \rightleftharpoons H_2CO_3$$

The increase in H_2CO_3 leads to a fall in pH. The tendency to acidosis is in part corrected by buffers other than bicarbonate/carbonic acid, and in this situation protein acts as a buffer in extracellular fluid, and haemoglobin, phosphate, and proteins within cells. A second compensatory mechanism is increased excretion of hydrogen ion by the kidneys.

13.5.2.2. Respiratory alkalosis. A decrease in CO_2 tension occurs when excretion of CO_2 by the lungs exceeds its production – *hypocapnia.* As production of CO_2 is constant respiratory alkalosis results from increased alveolar ventilation. This reduces P_{CO_2} and therefore H_2CO_3, leading to an increase in pH.

The alkalosis is in part corrected by a decrease in the production of HCO_3^- mainly within cells. A second compensatory mechanism is increased excretion of HCO_3^- in the urine.

It can be seen that acidosis or alkalosis, whether of metabolic or respiratory origin, is compensated rapidly by the buffering systems.

Metabolic abnormalities are also compensated more slowly by respiratory changes. Respiratory acidosis and alkalosis are compensated more slowly by renal mechanisms.

14. Osmotic diuresis

Solute cannot be excreted in the urine without water. In situations where it is necessary to excrete excess solute, water must be excreted with the solute. The need to excrete excess solute therefore leads to water depletion.

This is sometimes exploited therapeutically. Mannitol (a polyfructose molecule) is infused intravenously to produce an *osmotic diuresis.* It is filtered at the glomerulus but cannot be resorbed by the proximal renal tubules. Mannitol limits the resorption of water from the tubular lumen and leads to an increased volume of urine being excreted.

15. Free-water clearance

The glomerular filtrate consists of a mixture of solutes and water with the same osmolality as plasma, i.e., it is isotonic relative to plasma. When hypertonic urine (relative to plasma) is excreted it means that solute-free water has been resorbed by the renal tubules. When hypotonic urine (relative to plasma) is excreted it means that solute-free water has been excreted by the renal tubules. The volume of solute-free water which has been resorbed or excreted to change the urine from an isotonic filtrate to a hypertonic or hypotonic urine is known as the *free-water clearance* (C_{H_2O}).

For example, a daily solute load from the diet of about 600 millimoles has to be excreted. The maximum urine osmolality is 1200 mmol/kg H_2O and therefore the minimum urine volume in which 600 mmol of solute could be excreted is 500 ml. This urine volume is the minimum needed for osmolar clearance. If, however, the 24-hour urine is 1500 ml, then 500 ml can be regarded as the amount necessary for excretion of solute and 1000 ml as clearance of free water.

15.1. Effect of volume depletion in chronic renal failure

Patients with chronic impairment of renal function are unable to concentrate their urine maximally and in some the maximum possible concentration of urine is 300 mmol/kg H_2O or less. A urine volume of 2000 ml is therefore necessary to excrete the daily solute load of 600 mmol. Water is also needed for insensible loss via respiration and skin so that such a patient needs to ingest a minimum of 2500 ml water per day to remain in balance. If the patient becomes ill and cannot ingest fluids, or is deliberately deprived of fluid for intravenous pyelography or to test urinary concentrating power, severe volume depletion occurs.

Note, however, that some water is provided by metabolism as well as that ingested.

15.2. Polyuria

When the maximum urinary osmolality in chronic renal failure falls below 300 mmol/kg H_2O the urinary volume must exceed 3000 ml/24 hours to excrete the daily solute load.

The polyuria of chronic renal failure can be regarded as a form of nephrogenic diabetes insipidus (Chapter 9).

16. Antidiuretic hormone (ADH)

Antidiuretic hormone is an octapeptide, arginine vasopressin, which is secreted in the neurones of the supraoptic and paraventricular nuclei of the hypothalamus. It is transported along the neuronal axons to their endings within the posterior pituitary gland.

ADH is released from the posterior pituitary in response to elevation of plasma osmolality or plasma volume reduction. The immediate stimulus to the release of ADH appears to be dehydration of osmoreceptor cells within the brain. It is also released under situations of stress (emotion, fever, infections, operation, anaes-

14

thesia and analgesics). It is also produced by certain tumours (Chapter 10).

ADH increases the permeability of the renal distal tubules and collecting ducts to water. Under the action of ADH an increased amount of water is reabsorbed, with a corresponding increase in plasma volume, and a reduction in plasma osmolality. The urinary volume is reduced, with a corresponding increase in urinary osmolality.

Many drugs produce effects similar to excess ADH, e.g., chlorpropamide, cyclophosphamide, vincristine, clofibrate, barbiturates, indomethacin, and carbamazepine.

17. Aldosterone

Aldosterone is secreted by the zona glomerulosa of the adrenal cortex. It is secreted in response to a fall in blood volume, the change being sensed by the juxtaglomerular cells of the kidney. This is followed by the release of renin, which gives rise to the formation of angiotensin II which is carried to the adrenal glands and stimulates the secretion of aldosterone.

The secretion of aldosterone leads to retention of sodium and water with consequent increase in blood volume. When blood volume is restored the secretion of renin is inhibited again.

17.1. Hyperaldosteronism

Increased aldosterone secretion leads to elevated sodium retention and increased potassium excretion. The plasma potassium concentration is low and sodium concentration is normal or slightly elevated (Chapter 14). Increased aldosterone production may be primary (very rare) due to tumour or hyperplasia of the adrenal cortex (Conn's syndrome) or more commonly, secondary in association with congestive heart failure, severe hypertension, or cirrhosis.

17.2. Hyporeninaemic hypoaldosteronism

Decreased aldosterone secretion sometimes occurs in patients with a moderate degree of chronic renal failure in association with diabetes mellitus. This is due to damage to the juxta-glomerular apparatus leading to decreased secretion of renin and reduced production of aldosterone. Elevation of the plasma potassium out of proportion to the degree of renal failure is the characteristic feature. A similar situation may arise in some patients with interstitial nephritis.

2. The fluid compartments of the body

1. Fluid compartments of the body

Body fluid consists of an aqueous solution of salts, proteins and carbohydrates. Some of this solution is within cell membranes (intracellular fluid) and some is outside the membranes (extracellular fluid). Although differing in concentration of certain ions, especially sodium and potassium, the composition of the intracellular and extracellular fluids remains very constant in health. Fluid similar in composition to extracellular fluid circulates through the blood vessels and lymphatics, carrying the products of cell metabolism from their point of origin to their point of excretion through the lungs, liver, kidneys and bowel. All these organs are of course themselves made up of cells and extracellular fluid, and are themselves continuously contributing to and absorbing from the extracellular fluid.

As these three fluid compartments are closely interrelated, disorders of one compartment are quickly reflected in the other two compartments. Moreover, each disorder reacts on regulatory systems situated mainly within the brain and the vascular compartment.

About 60 per cent of body weight of the average adult male and 50 per cent of that of the average adult female, consists of water. The lower water content of the female body is due to its greater fat content, as fat contains less water than lean muscle. Thinner than average adults contain more water and fatter than average less water.

When the patient varies greatly on either side of the average the estimate of body water needs to be adjusted slightly (Table 3). Infants contain a considerably higher proportion of water than adults and are, therefore, particularly vulnerable to the effects of water loss (Table 3).

The intracellular fluid compartment contains two thirds of the body water. The remaining third is in the extracellular compartment, and of this third, one quarter is in the vascular space and three quarters in the intercellular space (Fig. 4). Water can pass readily between the vascular space and the intercellular space, and between the intracellular and extracellular spaces. Under normal circumstances the body is supplied with water principally by drinking but some is provided by internal metabolic processes. Water is lost from the body as urine, faecal water, sweat and via respiration.

Although the *percentage* of body weight which consists of water varies between males and females and between lean and fat subjects (Table 3), the *proportion* of

16

Table 3. Total body water as a percentage of body weight.

	Adult		Infant
	Male	Female	
Thin	65	55	80
Average	60	50	70
Fat	55	45	65

total body water in the intracellular and extracellular compartments remains unchanged.

An example of the fluid volumes in the body compartments of a female of average build weighing 60 kg is shown in Table 4. The important figure to be remembered is the total body water (30 l) as this figure is used in the calculation of the replacement of electrolyte deficiencies.

Table 4. Distribution of body water.
Average female weighing 60 kg.

Total body water:	50 per cent of 60	= 30 l
Intracellular water:	2/3 of 30 l	= 20 l
Extracellular water:	1/3 of 30 l	= 10 l
Intravascular water:	1/4 of 10 l	= 2.5 l

The fluid (whole blood) in the vascular compartment can be sampled easily. After separation of the cells from the plasma (or serum, i.e., plasma without fibrinogen) analysis for simple chemical composition is readily available in all hospital laboratories. Analysis of intracellular fluid composition is not usually carried out in hospital laboratories.

2. Composition of plasma and intracellular fluid

The average composition of plasma has been given in Table 1 and that of muscle cell in Table 2. The important differences in the concentrations of sodium and potassium should be noted, sodium being the predominant ion in plasma and potassium within cells. The exact composition assigned to muscle cell fluid varies with the method of preparation of the sample.

3. Role of the cell membrane pumps

The cell membrane pumps are responsible for the remarkable differences in the concentration of certain ions on either side of the cell membrane. The most

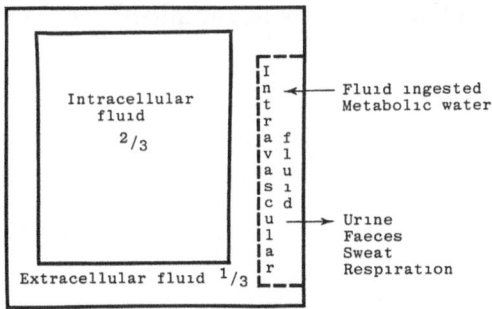

Fig. 4. The body fluid compartments.

important of these pumps are the sodium/potassium pump and the calcium/magnesium pump. The activity of the pumps seems to some extent regulated by changes in the intracellular ion concentration, for example the activity of the sodium/potassium pump decreases greatly when the intracellular sodium concentration falls to 10–20 mmol/l and is reactivated to remove sodium from the cell when the intracellular sodium concentration rises.

When cell pumps cease to function as a consequence of cell damage or anoxia enormous swelling of cells takes place because of the increased intracellular osmolality due to sodium diffusing into the cell. The cellular swelling may become great enough to burst the cell.

Although the concentrations of ions and other dissolved substances in the different fluid compartments differ, the total number of dissolved particles is equal in all compartments, as the osmolality depends on the number of particles in solution. If there is a change in osmolality in any one compartment, water moves from the adjacent compartment until a new osmotic equilibrium is reached.

It follows then that for the practical purpose of intravenous therapy, the differing concentrations of ions in the body compartments (due to the cell-membrane pumps) can be ignored. In any case it is not possible to exert any controlling influence on these regulatory mechanisms and intravenous therapy depends upon use of the simple laws of physical chemistry already described.

3. What can intravenous therapy accomplish?

1. Use of intravenous therapy

Intravenous therapy can be used to correct or prevent maladjustment of volume and of the concentrations of the more important ions in extracellular and intracellular fluid.

Abnormalities can arise three ways: (1) abnormal losses of body fluids; (3) abnormal retention of solutes or water normally excreted.

In general, only deficiencies arising from abnormal losses or from deficient replacements of normal losses can be corrected by intravenous therapy. At times it may be possible to achieve only partial correction of the abnormalities because there are certain limitations in the amount and type of fluid which may be given to the individual patient with safety. In certain circumstances intravenous therapy should not be attempted as it would lead to worsening rather than improvement in the patient's condition; for example correction of acidosis when the patient has left ventricular failure and is oedematous.

2. Limitations of intravenous therapy

The limitations to be observed are:

2.1. Limitation of volume

Factors which may limit the amount of volume which may be given include:

2.1.1. Amount of fluid loss
Unless there has been recent loss of fluid only a limited amount of intravenous fluid may be given. Fluid in excess of requirement may lead to left ventricular failure and pulmonary oedema.

2.1.2. Age
Elderly patients tolerate large fluid loads badly. In elderly patients it is better to err on the side of caution and give necessary fluids over a longer period than usual.

2.1.3. Cardiac and renal function
Impairment of either cardiac or renal function leads to impaired ability to excrete excess water.

2.1.4. Time
The volume which may be given with safety depends on the time over which it is administered.

2.1.5. Previous intravenous therapy
An attempt to correct an electrolyte disturbance may have been made already. The wrong type of fluid, or too much, may already have been given. This may make correction of the electrolyte disturbance unusually difficult.

3. Limitation of osmolality

The movement of water, followed by ions, between body compartments, which rapidly follows any direct addition of fluid to the vascular compartment, imposes a considerable limitation on judicious intravenous therapy. As mentioned in Chapter 1 water moves twice as fast as most ions and although a new equilibrium will later be established, the immediate effect is a change in osmolality. The direction of the change also needs to be taken into account.

The central nervous system is very sensitive to changes in osmolality. When osmolality is reduced by overloading with water, the hypothalamus reduces the production of antidiuretic hormone, and in health the excess water is quickly excreted by the kidneys. However, the sick patient may be unable to excrete the excess water because of poor cardiac or renal function, and left ventricular failure will result.

A very rapid increase in vascular and therefore extracellular osmolality leads to rapid withdrawal of fluid from cells. In the brain this may lead to shrinkage of cells which may be severe enough to tear small cerebral blood vessels causing petechial haemorrhages and sometimes irreparable damage to the brain.

4. Limitation of sodium

The osmolality of the extracellular fluid is largely due to the presence of sodium ions. The relative contribution of the various cations and anions in plasma is shown in Table 5. Sodium contributes no less than 140 milliosmoles per kg, compared with the 144 milliosmoles contributed by all the anions, and with 2 by plasma proteins and 5 each by glucose and urea. Under abnormal circumstances an elevated concentration of glucose or urea can increase plasma osmolality substantially and produce a hyperosmolar state.

Table 5. The contribution of ions and molecules to plasma osmolality.

	mosmol/kg
Sodium	140
Potassium	4
Anions chloride	
bicarbonate	
phosphate	144
sulphate	
organic acids	
Proteins	2
Urea	5
Glucose	5
Total	300

Within the cells potassium is the predominant ion (Table 2) and makes the largest contribution to intracellular osmolality.

The overwhelming importance of sodium in the regulation of the osmolality of plasma and extracellular fluid means that sodium-containing solutions must be used with care.

If sodium is given in amounts sufficient to raise the plasma sodium to 160 mmol/l or above, muscle twitching, mental confusion, convulsions and eventually coma ensue. The effect of the excess sodium is more marked when the concentration of sodium is raised very rapidly. The mortality associated with hypernatraemia is high, and if the patient survives there may be permanent brain damage.

Neurological disturbance occurs with hypernatraemia of any cause, but the most serious consequences arise when the hypernatraemia develops rapidly.

4.1. Sodium space

The concept of 'sodium space' is a useful safeguard against inadvertent production of hypernatraemia during electrolyte infusion. When a sodium space is present there is a deficit in body sodium due to excessive loss or deficient intake. There is a reduction in plasma sodium concentration which is *not* due to overhydration. When a sodium space is present the electrolyte disturbance can be corrected without risk of production of hypernatraemia. When a sodium space is not present, care is needed in prescribing sodium.

The 'sodium space' is the shortfall of the plasma sodium concentration below the normal level of 140 mmol/l (i.e., 140 − observed plasma sodium concentration in mmol/l) multiplied by the estimated volume of total body water. It might be thought that as sodium resides almost entirely within the extracellular compartment the volume used for the calculation should be that of the extracellular space. However, when sodium is either added to or subtracted from the extracellular compartment, by its osmotic effect it causes a shift of water between cells and extracellular fluid. thus the osmotic effect of sodium is distributed throughout the entire volume of body water and it is this volume which must be taken into account when replacing any deficiency.

For a woman weighing 60 kg with a plasma sodium level of 130 mmol/l the 'sodium space' is therefore:

$$(140 - 130) \times 30 = 300 \, \text{mmol}$$

30 litres being 50% of her body weight in kg (assuming that she is of average build, neither lean nor fat).

A serious anion abnormality, usually acidosis, may be present in a patient lacking a 'sodium space'. In this situation only a very limited amount of sodium-containing electrolyte may be given over a short time period. Provided there is continuing urinary excretion of sodium or a loss by other routes, this can be exploited to allow for the gradual correction of the anion abnormality. If the patient is acidotic an amount of sodium equivalent to the previous day's losses may be given daily as sodium bicarbonate.

5. Limitation of hydrogen ion concentration

The need to maintain the body fluids within the narrow range of physiological pH must be taken into account when prescribing intravenous therapy.

The importance of the bicarbonate/carbonic buffer system for the maintenance of extracellular pH has already been noted. In situations where there is a deficiency or relative deficiency of bicarbonate it is important to give bicarbonate *first* to replete the buffering power of plasma. It is particularly important to remember this when there is little or no 'sodium space', when all permissible sodium should be given as sodium bicarbonate.

The importance of haemoglobin as a buffer is sometimes overlooked. In anaemic subjects its lack contributes to their greater tendency to become acidotic.

5.1. Respiratory acidosis/alkalosis

Respiration plays an important part in the regulation of tissue pH, via the bicarbonate/carbonic acid buffer system of extracellular fluid. The end product of many metabolic processes is carbon dioxide and water.

$$CO_2 + H_2O \rightleftharpoons H_2CO_3 \rightleftharpoons HCO_3^- + H^+$$

Failure of adequate ventilation by the lungs leads to retention of carbon dioxide, formation of carbonic acid, which in turn produces bicarbonate and hydrogen ion, i.e., *respiratory acidosis* (Chapter 18).

Increased ventilation leads to excessive loss of carbon dioxide and consumption of H ion with formation of hydroxyl molecules, i.e., *respiratory alkalosis* (Chapter 18).

Acidosis of respiratory origin cannot be treated with intravenous infusion of sodium bicarbonate. The treatment is the correction of the abnormality of respiration if this is possible.

5.2. Metabolic acidosis

The metabolic processes of cells result in the production of hydrogen ions and the formation of acidic waste products. Some hydrogen ion is ingested in food. The main route for disposal of hydrogen ion is the kidney, the mechanism has been described already in Chapter 1.

Metabolic acidosis may be caused by:

5.2.1
Kidney failure with retention of hydrogen ion. It is often unwise to attempt to correct metabolic acidosis due to renal failure by giving sodium bicarbonate. If the patient has hypertension or oedema, both may be made worse by giving sodium bicarbonate, and the acidosis can be corrected safely only by dialysis.

5.2.2
Renal tubular acidosis which is due to deficient resorption of sodium bicarbonate and/or to deficient excretion of hydrogen ion by the renal tubules.

5.2.3
Increased production of acid, for example keto-acidosis associated with hyperglycaemia in uncontrolled diabetes mellitus.

5.2.4
Loss of bicarbonate from the gastrointestinal tract in diarrhoea, or in bile.

Sodium bicarbonate can be given safely in renal tubular acidosis, in keto-acidosis and after diarrhoea, as sodium loss in urine continues and there is no danger of sodium overload.

5.3. Metabolic alkalosis

Metabolic alkalosis may result from loss of the hydrogen ion in gastric juice by vomiting or by nasogastric aspiration. This abnormality is very suitable for correction by intravenous therapy, as there is ample 'space' for sodium and water. There has been loss of both sodium and water, as well as hydrogen ion in the vomitus.

Alkalosis may result from excessive ingestion of sodium bicarbonate, usually self-administered for the relief of dyspepsia. The treatment is cessation of ingestion of sodium bicarbonate, not intravenous therapy.

6. Potassium deficiency

Potassium deficiency occurs in a wide variety of clinical situations (Chapter 15).

The normal plasma potassium level is 3.5–5.0 mmol/l. When the plasma concentration falls below 2.5 mmol/l muscle weakness appears, sometimes accompanied by paraesthesia or pain in muscles. This may progress to paralysis, most prominent in the legs, later affecting the respiratory muscles. The kidneys fail to concentrate urine normally and polyuria and thirst develop. Later oliguria occurs and the plasma urea rises.

Since potassium is the predominant intracellular cation the amount needed to correct deficiency cannot be determined by any fixed formula. Deficiency causing symptoms may vary from 250 to 1000 mmol. Potassium deficiency can often be corrected by mouth, but large deficits may require weeks for correction.

Potassium can be given intravenously but must be administered in dilute solution (diluted in 5% dextrose or dextrose in saline). The rate of infusion should not ordinarily exceed 20 mmol/hr. Rapid infusion of potassium chloride in a patient who is over-digitalized may cause ventricular arrhythmias, and must be avoided. It is usually given in concentrations of 20–50 mmol/l. Where there is a volume restriction with severe potassium deficiency concentrations of up to 80 mmol/l may be required, but such high concentrations must be given slowly, and ECG monitoring is desirable.

It is sometimes stated that potassium should not be given intravenously unless the urinary output is 'adequate'. However, oliguria may be present when the patient has serious potassium deficiency, e.g., following prolonged vomiting or nasogastric aspiration. Intravenous infusion of sodium chloride solution without potassium does not correct this abnormality, but rapid improvement in urinary output follows intravenous administration of potassium chloride diluted in sodium chloride solution. The urinary output should be carefully charted and the serum electrolytes assessed after 12 hours in these circumstances.

Finally it is never essential to fully correct an electrolyte abnormality immediately. Partial correction usually leads to considerable improvement in the patient's clinical condition, even though the biochemical evidence of improvement may be disappointing. It is always safer to under-correct than to over-correct an electrolyte abnormality, especially if the patient is old and may have poor cardiac reserve. Further correction can follow during the second and subsequent 24 hours.

4. The clinical history

The importance of obtaining a careful history of the onset of the illness leading to the electrolyte upset cannot be over emphasised. Most electrolyte disturbances which can be corrected by intravenous therapy arise as a result of either abnormal losses of body fluids or of deficient replacement of normal losses. The history often reveals the cause of the illness and provides important clues to the type of biochemical abnormality present. The laboratory results should serve merely as confirmation and as a guide to the degree of abnormality to be corrected. Indeed, if the laboratory results are not in keeping with the clinical history, the laboratory tests should be repeated in case a laboratory error has occurred.

Electrolyte disturbances of which the causation cannot be identified from the history are comparatively rare though it is essential to be aware of them. The rarer causes will be discussed in later chapters.

The clinical history gives important clues to the causes of electrolyte disturbance (Table 6).

1. Deficient intake

Deficient intake of water and electrolytes occurs most commonly in infancy and in old age. In the presence of continuing urinary and faecal losses it eventually leads to dehydration and electrolyte depletion. Elderly people living alone are particularly vulnerable, but even in hospital the elderly patient may become depleted. An elderly patient with a fractured neck of femur or other orthopaedic condition requiring treatment on a gantry may be unable to reach fluids on the bedside locker, and become too confused to ask for help. The experienced ward sister often guards against this possibility by an informal fluid balance chart on which is recorded the amount of fluid actually taken, as opposed to what is left available on the locker.

2. Vomiting or aspiration

The commonest cause of serious water and electrolyte loss is vomiting. Patients vomit at home, vomiting may continue after admission to hospital, but if it is severe gastric aspiration is then commenced.

Table 6. Causes of fluid and electrolyte imbalance.

1.	Deficient intake
2.	Vomiting or aspiration of gastric fluid
3.	Loss from gastrointestinal fistula
4.	Biliary loss
5.	Diarrhoea
6.	Excessive urinary loss
7.	Impaired renal function
8.	Following operation of urinary diversion
9.	Excessive sweat loss
10.	Drugs
11.	Electrolyte disturbances associated with intravenous therapy

When vomiting occurs at home precise information about the amount is seldom available. It is worth obtaining as accurate information as possible about the total duration of vomiting, the number of times per 24 hours it has occurred, and whether the patient has been able to retain any fluid between the vomits. Information about urinary output is useful – if the patient has noticed that urine has become scanty it is evidence of serious deficiency. After admission to hospital a fluid balance chart should record all fluids lost and taken (Chapter 6). Vomitus is often not measured, even in hospital, because considerable amounts may be lost over bedclothes or estimates may be recorded instead of actual measured amounts.

Serious disturbances occasionally arise as a result of deliberate vomiting with or without deficient intake. I recall two patients with severe electrolyte disturbances typical of chronic vomiting, although neither gave any history of vomiting and appeared to eat extremely well when in hospital. Although the cause was suspected, it was some time before these patients were caught in the act of self-induced vomiting. A somewhat similar disturbance occurred in a prisoner who went on hunger and thirst strike for ten days after which he consented to take fluids but refused solids. Advice was requested because after 30 days the blood urea began to rise and it was noted that he had marked depletion of potassium. On attempting to get him to take potassium by mouth he began to vomit, no doubt deliberately. He successfully resisted attempts to correct his electrolyte abnormality by the oral route in the prison sick bay (by pretence of compliance and disposing of his tablets down his wash hand basin) and refused intravenous therapy in the security wing of a hospital. He was transferred to an ordinary hospital ward under guard but he escaped. When re-captured a year later his electrolytes and urea were normal. This time he knew the routine and quickly vomited his way back to his electrolyte problem and depressed renal function.

26

Table 7. Electrolyte content of gastrointestinal fluids.

	Electrolyte concentrations (mmol/l)			
	Sodium	Potassium	Bicarbonate	Chloride
Gastric	40– 80	5–15	0	125
Bile	140–160	0–10	40	100
Pancreas	130–150	0–10	100	70
Small bowel	80–140	0–10	30	100
Ileostomy	120–140	15–20	30	100
Cecostomy	60–100	15–30	10	40

3. Loss from gastrointestinal fistulae

The volume of fluid lost is greater the higher the level of the fistula. Loss from a fistula into dressings is often not recorded on the fluid balance chart, but can be measured by weighing dressings before and after use, or by attaching an ileostomy bag to the area of the fistula. The electrolyte content of gastrointestinal fluid from different levels is shown in Table 7.

4. Loss of bile

Loss of bile may also occur into dressings and remain unrecorded.

5. Diarrhoea

Diarrhoea is an important cause of electrolyte disturbance, especially in the very young, the elderly and in the third world. Diarrhoea is frequently encountered amongst tourists, but as it is usually of brief duration electrolyte therapy is seldom needed. It is useful to enquire about the duration of the diarrhoea, the frequency, quantity and quality of bowel motions.

The electrolyte content of diarrhoeal fluid is very variable. The most severe losses are associated with infection by the *Vibrio cholerae*.

Occasionally a serious deficiency of potassium may result from chronic abuse of purgatives, which the patient usually does not mention. The history should always include information on bowel habit, including use of laxatives.

6. Excessive urinary loss

Electrolyte disturbance due to excessive urinary losses sometimes arises over a considerable period. Excessive urinary volume may have been present for so long that the patient regards it as normal and does not mention it. It may be a result of diuretic therapy for hypertension or of impairment of renal function by disease. Excessive loss of water and electrolytes often follows relief of urinary obstruction, due to impaired renal tubular function. Losses following relief of obstruction can be very large and it is essential to replace them completely until renal tubular function improves and urinary concentrating power recovers.

7. Impaired renal function

A history of renal disease of any type, at any time in the past, should alert to the possibility of residual impairment of renal function. Chronic renal disease may remain undiscovered until the increased metabolic load associated with an acute illness reveals impaired excretion of waste products.

Impaired renal function may be suggested by a history of either excessively large or excessively scanty urinary output. It may be responsible for excessive loss of sodium, or of potassium, or for failure to excrete sodium or potassium leading to hypernatraemia or hyperkalaemia. Impaired renal function may lead to excessive loss of water or to overhydration.

8. Urinary diversion operations

Diversion of the ureters may be required in patients with disease of the distal urinary tract or pelvis. Diversion of the urine into the sigmoid colon may be complicated by severe hyperchloraemic acidosis with hypokalaemia. This may occur within a few days or weeks of the operation, or not until years later.

The use of the colon as a reservoir for urine results in increased loss of bicarbonate and potassium and absorption of chloride. Tubular reabsorption of chloride probably also contributes to the hyperchloraemia. The biochemical abnormality is metabolic acidosis with a normal anion gap. Regurgitation of urine mixed with faeces into the ureters leads to repeated episodes of pyelonephritis, and eventually to impairment in renal tubular function and worsening of the biochemical abnormality.

Although this complication has been recognised for many years, urinary diversion into the sigmoid colon is still used in patients with neoplastic disease of the bladder whose prognosis is thought to be poor. Patients are still encountered in whom this operation was carried out 20 to 30 years ago for ectopia vesica.

The problem is less when an isolated loop of ileum is used for the urinary diversion. The loop should be short and serve merely as a conduit to lead urine into a bag outside the body. If the loop is large enough to act as a reservoir for urine, bicarbonate is lost and hyperchloraemic acidosis develops as with a ureterosigmoidostomy.

9. Excessive loss of sweat

Sweat contains 40–80 mmol of sodium and 0–5 mmol of potassium per litre. Excessive sweating usually accompanies febrile illnesses. The amount of fluid lost as sweat can be estimated by weighing clothing and bedding before and after use but this is seldom done and an estimate has to suffice. About 250 ml *additional* water is lost via sweating and increased respiratory loss for each 1°C rise in temperature.

Excessive sweating may occur during work carried out in abnormally hot environments such as tropical conditions, and in ships' boiler rooms. Under these circumstances the loss of sodium becomes significant and extra salt is needed.

10. Drug-induced electrolyte disturbances

A careful history of all drugs taken before the onset of illness can be very helpful. Apart from the obvious importance of diuretics and laxatives, mentioned already, many other drugs can cause electrolyte disturbances. Table 8 lists some of the commoner drugs which may cause electrolyte disturbances.

Table 8. Drugs which may cause electrolyte disturbances.

---

1. *Drugs causing sodium and water retention* (oedema, left ventricular failure, hypertension)
   Corticosteroids, especially fludrocortisone
   Corticotrophin
   Oestrogens
   Stilboestrol
   Non-steroid anti-inflammatory drugs, especially phenylbutazone
   Many blood-pressure lowering drugs, especially minoxidil and diazoxide
   Vasodilators
   Carbenoxolone
   Diuretics (after cessation)
2. *Sodium-containing drugs*
   Sodium bicarbonate
   Antacid preparations
   Andrew's Liver Salts and Eno's Fruit Salts
   Antibiotics especially carbenicillin
   X-ray contrast media
3. *Drug-induced sodium loss*
   Barbiturates
   Tricyclic antidepressants

Table 8. Continued.

    Anaesthetic drugs
    Clofibrate
    Chlorpropamide
    Diuretics
4. *Potassium elevation*
    Potassium chloride 'substitute salt' (Selora)
    Potassium-sparing diuretics
    Clavulanic acid (potassium salt; combined with amoxycillin in Augmentin)
    Fruit juice
    Instant coffee
    Chocolate drinks
5. *Potassium loss*
    Corticosteroids
    Carbenoxolone
    Liquorice (glycyrrhic acid)
    Diuretics
    Laxatives
    Enemas
6. *Drugs causing water retention*
    Nicotine
    Chlorpropamide
    Cyclophosphamide
    Vincristine
    Clofibrate
    Barbariturates
    Morphine
    Carbamazepine
    Indomethacin
    Isoproterenol
7. *Drugs causing water loss*
    Diuretics
    Lithium
8. *Metabolic acidosis*
    Salicylate
    Ethanol
    Methanol
    Paraldehyde
    Ethylene glycol
    Vitamin D excess
    Out-dated tetracycline
    Ammonium chloride
    Acetazolamide
    Ion exchange resins
    Phenformin
    Isoniazid (overdose)
9. *Metabolic alkalosis*
    Sodium bicarbonate
    Diuretics
    Carbenoxolone
    Liquorice

10.1

Fludrocortisone is usually given for the purpose of replacing aldosterone in the treatment of adreno-cortical failure, but the retention of sodium and water is an undesirable side effect of the other drugs listed. A rise in blood pressure accompanies the retention of sodium and water when corticosteroids and oestrogens are given. Many hypotensive drugs, especially minoxidil and diazoxide, but also other vasodilators including hydrallazine, beta-blockers and occasionally reserpine and methyldopa cause sodium and water retention. Oedema may complicate the use of any of these drugs and can be very severe with minoxidil and diazoxide (both vasodilators), especially when renal function is impaired. A diuretic drug should be given along with minoxidil and diazoxide.

It may seem surprising that diuretics can cause oedema, but when these are used for long periods compensatory mechanisms lead to retention of sodium and water. If the diuretic is discontinued the compensatory mechanisms persist for several days after the diuretic effect has disappeared, and oedema may develop.

10.2

Some drugs contain sodium in considerable amount. Apart from sodium bicarbonate itself, all antacids contain sodium, including magnesium trisilicate preparations and 'coating preparations' (e.g., Gaviscon).

The sodium content of some X-ray contrast media is considerable. These are sometimes used for high-dose pyelography, e.g., Conray-420 may contain as much as 172 mmol of sodium per 150 ml. The sodium dose can be reduced by using a meglumine-based contrast medium for at least part of the dose. All these drugs may cause oedema, and in susceptible subjects, hypertension and left ventricular failure.

10.3

Some drugs increase renal loss of sodium, diuretics being given for this purpose. However, the prolonged use of diuretics leads to compensatory retention of sodium and water which continues for a few days after the drug is discontinued.

10.4

Patients who have been told to keep their sodium intake low may use 'substitute salt' which is usually potassium chloride. If renal failure is present they may rapidly develop hyperkalaemia. Potassium-sparing diuretics such as spironolactone, triamterene and amiloride may cause hyperkalaemia in patients with poor renal function.

10.5

Carbenoxolone can cause profound potassium deficiency because of a mineral corticoid-like effect on the distal renal tubules. The active principle in liquorice, glycyrrhic acid, chemically resembles aldosterone and like it causes increased potassium excretion. Regular use of laxatives may cause chronic hypokalaemia which may lead to impaired renal function. Patients often do not inform their doctor that they take laxatives and it is worth making a regular practice of asking whether they are taken. Some potassium is lost in enemas but these are not often used repeatedly, and are unlikely to cause significant potassium deficiency.

10.6

Many drugs cause water retention. Nicotine causes water retention by stimulating release of ADH, and clofibrate, vincristine and isoproterenol may act in the same way. Indomethacin, and possibly chlorpropamide enhance the action of vasopressin.

Little is known about the mode of action of the other drugs causing water retention.

10.7

Lithium, as well as diuretics, causes excessive urinary loss of water.

10.8

Drugs which cause acidosis are particularly likely to do so in patients with impaired renal function – for example, regular use of normal therapeutic doses of salicylates may occasionally lead to severe acidosis in such patients. Methanol was the cause of extreme acidosis in an elderly man who had imbibed home-made poteen. He did not have renal failure or hyperglycaemia. He admitted to alcoholism but denied taking any unusual drink until his eyesight began to fail rapidly.

Acetazolamide given for the treatment of glaucoma or tinnitus can cause severe acidosis in elderly patients with impairment of renal function.

11. Electrolyte disturbances associated with intravenous therapy

Electrolyte disturbances arising in patients who have already been treated with intravenous therapy for days or weeks can pose difficult problems. A careful study of the case notes and fluid balance and drug records usually reveals how the disturbance has occurred. The commonest errors are to give insufficient potassium, or failure to account for all fluids and sodium lost or given.

12. Thirst

The conscious patient may complain of thirst. In the context of the patient with a possible electrolyte disturbance thirst may be regarded as a sign as well as a symptom.

The physiology of thirst is complicated and imperfectly understood. In normal circumstances thirst occurs in response to water loss and the drinking of water abolishes it in a satisfying way. Thirst is induced also by eating salty food or by intravenous infusion of hypertonic saline. Infusion of other solutes such as sorbitol, sodium sulphate and sodium acetate also produces thirst. Sodium salts, which effectively remain in the extracellular compartment, and therefore withdraw water from cells, are more effective producers of thirst than urea which diffuses readily into cells. These facts suggest that thirst is a response to intracellular dehydration, but patients may sometimes complain of thirst when their plasma sodium is low rather than raised. Thirst sometimes occurs also with potassium depletion, which perhaps may be explained by secondary loss of water from cells because of polyuria associated with potassium deficiency. Therefore, thirst may be associated with water depletion, sodium overload, sodium depletion, potassium depletion and also sometimes with congestive heart failure.

Thirst may be due to local factors such as dryness of the mouth due to diminished salivation, e.g., in Sjögren's syndrome.

The very ill patient may not be aware of thirst despite adequate reasons for its presence. The presence or absence of thirst is therefore often not very helpful as a clue to the cause of a electrolyte problem.

13. Dyspnoea

Breathlessness may be due to acute or chronic pulmonary diseases, cardiac disease or sodium and water overload with acute pulmonary oedema. Severe dyspnoea of sudden onset, with cough and copious frothy sputum, is suggestive of pulmonary oedema. The sputum may be blood-stained.

A comprehensive and accurate case history is the first step towards good electrolyte management.

5. Physical examination of the patient

Electrolyte disturbances may arise as a result of disease or trauma affecting any system of the body. The physical signs of fluid and electrolyte disturbance may be numerous or surprisingly few and may be overshadowed by the causative disease. However certain points are specially relevant (Table 9).

1. Weight

An effort should be made to weigh the patient, preferably in kilograms. It may be impossible to weigh the very ill patient unless bed scales are available, but if they are available it is very helpful to arrange for the patient to be weighed daily as a clear indication of the state of hydration.

In the absence of facilities for weighing, the conscious patient may know his recent weight or his weight when at his prime, i.e., his lean weight. The total body water is estimated as 60 per cent of weight in kg in males, and 50 per cent of weight in females (Chapter 2).

Table 9. Physical examination.

---

 1. Weight
 2. Temperature
 3. Skin
 4. Sweating
 5. Mucous membranes
 6. Oedema
 7. Jugular venous pressure
 8. Blood pressure
 9. Hypotension
10. Hypertension
11. Cardiac assessment
12. Lungs
13. Anaemia
14. Abdomen
15. Tendon reflexes
16. Restless patient
17. Fontanelle in infancy

---

2. Temperature

Increase in body temperature is associated with increased loss of water through sweating and respiration. The cause of the rise in temperature is important, as if as is usually the case, it is due to infection, there will be an associated increase in catabolism and a greater production of nitrogenous and acidic waste products, as well as potassium, from breakdown of cells. Moreover, severe infection may cause hypotension with reduction in urine volume and failure to excrete the products of catabolism. A blood culture is an essential investigation in all such patients, especially if hypotension accompanies the rise in temperature.

3. Skin

The skin should be inspected for pigmentation. The pigmentation of jaundice may vary from pale yellow to greenish bronze. Chronic renal failure may cause a pale to deep brownish coloration, Addison's disease a brownish pigmentation which is present also in the mouth.

The condition of the skin provides important clues about the state of water balance, and about the state of combined balance of sodium and water (Table 10).

The presence or absence of visible sweat should be noted.

When marked loss of water has occurred the skin feels warm and dry, including the axilla and groin areas.

When excess water is present (without excess sodium) the skin feels warm and moist. There may be oedema of skin, which can be demonstrated by the production of a fingerprint when the finger is rolled over an area of subcutaneous bone.

The turgor of the skin gives information about the state of balance of both water and sodium. This is assessed by picking up a fold of the skin between the finger and thumb and then releasing it. Skin turgor can be assessed conveniently on the front of the chest wall below the clavicle where the skin is slightly loose. The fold picked up must not include subcutaneous tissue. In the water-and-salt-depleted patient the skin fold persists for an appreciable time. By the time this sign is present the adult patient is short of at least 3 litres of volume, and the longer the fold persists the greater is the deficiency.

The inexperienced observer may confuse wasting with loss of skin turgor. Turgor

Table 10. Condition of the skin.

Warm and dry:	water loss
Warm and moist:	water excess
Persistent skin fold:	water and sodium loss
Pitting oedema:	water and sodium excess

or its lack relates to the skin, wasting relates to the underlying subcutaneous tissue. The characteristic of wasting is a general looseness of the skin over the body and this is often most easily appreciated on the abdomen. Wasting and loss of skin turgor may be present together, for example, in the patient with chronic vomiting associated with disease of the upper gastrointestinal tract.

In a child who is depleted of sodium and water the face as a whole looks shrunken, the skin appears tightly stretched over the skull and the eyeballs are sunken into their sockets. A sunken facies in an adult is more likely to result from wasting of subcutaneous tissue than from dehydration.

The *ocular tension* is reduced when marked volume depletion has occurred. This is assessed by gentle pressure on the eyeball with the lid closed. The tension of one's own eyeball acts as a convenient control. Eyeball tension is reduced only when considerable depletion has occurred.

4. Sweating

The presence of visible sweat indicates that the patient has a greater than normal loss of fluid via the skin. It follows that the usual allowance of fluid for insensible loss via the skin and respiration will need to be increased.

In a patient who is unconscious, sweating may be due to hypoglycaemia and the blood sugar should be estimated urgently. A dexrostix test can be done in the ward while awaiting the laboratory result. The other classical signs of hypoglycaemia such as dilated pupils and tachycardia are not always present. If in doubt, dextrose should be given intravenously while awaiting the result of the blood test.

5. Mucous membranes

The tongue and mucous membranes of an underhydrated patient appear dry and shrunken. Sometimes the mouth and tongue may be dry because of mouth-breathing, rather than because of underhydration. In these circumstances other signs of underhydration are absent. Inspection of the conjunctiva may suggest anaemia, which may be a clue to chronically impaired renal function. Pigmentation of the oral mucosa suggests Addison's disease.

6. Oedema

Retention of sodium and water leads to the formation of oedema. This is expansion of the subcutaneous tissues which becomes visible as swelling. The swelling can characteristically be dented by firm pressure with the finger or thumb – pitting oedema, the pit remaining for some time after the pressure is removed (Fig. 5).

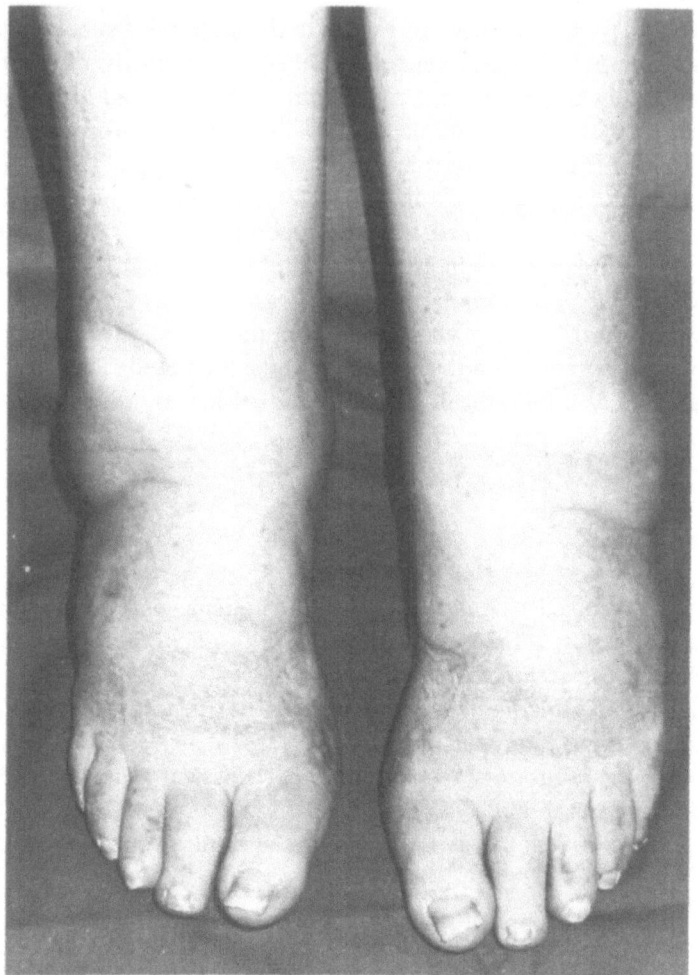

Fig. 5. Pitting oedema in dependent areas.
Photograph courtsey of Dr J. F. Douglas.

If the patient has not been confined to bed, the first sign may be slight ankle oedema. In the bed-ridden patient oedema first appears on the under (dorsal) side of the thighs (Fig. 6) and later in the lumbosacral area. In gross overload there is pitting oedema of the abdominal wall.

Oedema of one limb or one part of the body is not due to overload with sodium and water. A local cause such as lymphatic obstruction should be sought. Lymphatic oedema does not pit on pressure.

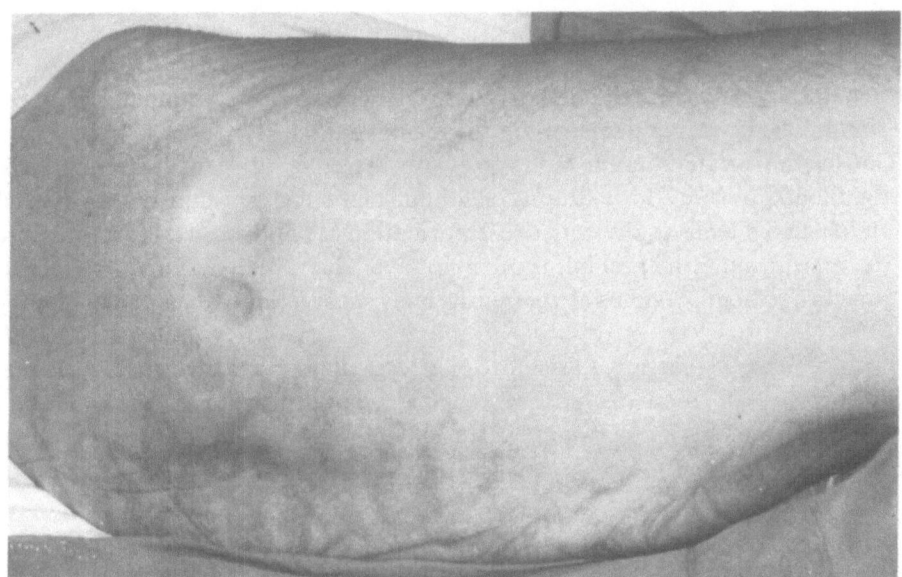

Fig. 6. Pitting oedema of thigh in recumbent patient.

7. Jugular venous pressure

When gross overload with sodium and water is present there is an increase in the circulating blood volume and the symptoms and signs are indistinguishable from those of heart failure. The neck veins communicate directly with the right atrium and changes in the mean pressure within them, and the pulsations occurring with each cardiac cycle, reflect the mean atrial pressure and pressure changes during the cardiac cycle.

The root of the neck is inspected when the patient is lying comfortably in semi-recumbent position (45°), the head being supported by appropriate pillows. Under normal circumstances there should be no visible filling of the neck veins but some slight pulsation may be visible. Venous filling, if present, is estimated as cm above the manubrium, and in extreme cases can approach the angle of the jaw. The pressure in the neck veins may also be raised because of partial obstruction between them and the atrium, for example, by a tumour, but pulsations are absent.

The jugular venous pressure may be elevated due to cardiac defeat but in these circumstances some degree of sodium and water overload may be present and indeed is often the precipitating cause of cardiac failure. Triple rhythm and basal lung crepitations are additional signs of cardiac defeat.

8. Blood pressure

Ideally the blood pressure should be recorded in both the erect and supine positions, but in ill patients the measurement in the recumbent position must suffice.

Considerable variations in blood pressure are compatible with normal well-being. Blood pressure is lower during childhood and pregnancy than during normal adult life, and it tends to rise with age. Information about the usual blood pressure of the patient can be helpful but is often not available. A fall in blood pressure to normal in a patient previously hypertensive may cause a rapid reduction in urinary output.

Change in blood pressure is therefore of greater significance than absolute levels. Quite low levels of blood pressure, if associated with warm well-perfused hands and feet, are often compatible with good perfusion of the kidneys and adequate production of urine.

9. Hypotension

Any serious reduction in blood pressure leads to a fall in glomerular filtration rate and urine volume, which leads to failure of excretion of water, electrolytes and metabolic waste products. When the urinary volume is low the constraints of fluid volume and sodium 'space' become limiting factors for intravenous fluid prescription. It is, therefore, very important to discover the cause of the hypotension and rectify it as soon as possible.

Common causes of hypotension are listed in Table 11.

Table 11. Causes of hypotension.

1. Hypovolaemia
1.1.   Blood loss
1.2.   Plasma loss
1.3.   Severe water and electrolyte depletion
2. Bacteraemia
3. Myocardial infarction
4. Over-administration of hypotensive drugs
5. Acute adrenocortical insufficiency
6. Cardiac tamponade
7. Cardiac arrythmia
8. Pulmonary embolism

9.1. Hypovolaemia

A sudden fall in blood volume from any cause leads to hypotension.

9.1.1

Blood loss is a common cause of hypovolaemia. A fall in blood pressure accompanied by tachycardia without a rise in temperature is suggestive of blood loss. External loss of blood should be obvious but considerable loss may occur under dressings without anyone noticing it. Internal bleeding may be considerable before it is suspected. Large losses may occur suddenly into the abdomen from rupture of the spleen, a tear in the liver, or a ruptured aneurysm and the situation may become catastrophic within a few minutes. The slow loss of blood into the retro-peritoneal space is more difficult to diagnose and is suggested by increasing anaemia accompanying hypotension and tachycardia. Serial measurements of abdominal girth are sometimes useful. Bleeding from an acute peptic ulcer or from gastric erosions is a common cause of blood loss in severely ill patients. There may be vomiting of blood, or blood may suddenly appear in the gastric aspirate. Sometimes the first indication of upper gastrointestinal bleeding may be the passage of a large tarry motion. Serial measurements of haemaglobin and testing of faeces for occult blood are useful when slow blood loss is suspected.

9.1.2

Loss of plasma into a large area of venous obstruction, such as a limb, an area of extensive operative dissection, or a burned area may cause hypovolaemia. During the development of paralytic ileus sequestration of extracellular fluid into dilated bowel loops occurs. These losses are sometimes referred to as 'third space' losses.

9.1.3

Severe water and electrolyte depletion may cause hypotension. Peripheral circulatory failure, with cold extremities and sluggish circulation, is usually present.

9.2. Bacteraemia

This is a common cause of hypotension in severely injured patients, and after operations and anaesthesia. It may occur during intravenous therapy for treatment of medical conditions such as diabetic coma. The diagnosis is obvious when the patient has a rigor followed by a high temperature, as well as hypotension. However, rigors may be absent and the fall in blood pressure may precede the rise in temperature. In the very ill patient the temperature may not rise at all. Blood cultures are essential if bacteraemia is suspected.

9.3. Myocardial infarction

Hypotension due to myocardial infarction occurs surprisingly often in patients seriously ill from other causes. Chest pain may or may not be present, and if present needs to be differentiated from that due to a pulmonary embolus. An ECG, chest X-ray and estimation of cardiac enzymes are needed.

9.4. Hypotensive drugs

Over-administration of hypotensive drugs is especially likely during the early phase of bringing hypertension under control, but can lead to hypotension at any time. Postural hypotension (i.e., a fall in blood pressure on changing from supine to erect position) may be an early sign of volume depletion as well as evidence of over control of hypertension.

A patient already stabilised on hypotensive therapy usually requires less drugs after operation and anaesthesia. Hypotensive drugs should be given in reduced dosage, or even omitted, for a few days after operation.

9.5. Adrenocortical insufficiency

Acute adrenocortical insufficiency should be considered if hypotension occurs in a patient who has been receiving long-term corticosteroid therapy for any reason, especially if it has been given in divided doses rather than as a single early morning dose, or who has had an adrenalectomy or hypophysectomy. Weakness, nausea, vomiting and abdominal pain may precede the development of hypotension.

Hypotensive crisis occurs in Addison's disease where the brownish grey pigmentation of the skin and mucous membranes provides a clue. Destruction of the adrenals by tuberculosis was formerly the commonest cause of Addison's disease. Acute adrenal crisis may result from haemorrhage into the adrenals in meningococcal septicaemia (Waterhouse-Friderichsen's syndrome).

9.6. Cardiac tamponade

A large pericardial effusion or haemorrhage is a fairly uncommon cause of hypotension, but can occur very rapidly.

9.7. Cardiac arrhythmia

This may lead to hypotension. Auscultation and ECG should suggest the cause.

9.8. Pulmonary embolism

This has already been mentioned as a cause of hypotension, in the differential diagnosis of myocardial infarction. The legs should be examined for a possible source of emboli in a patient who has had recent surgery, especially pelvic surgery, and other sources of emboli considered. Besides a chest X-ray and ECG, a lung scan may be very helpful.

If no adequate explanation of hypotension can be found, it is wise to take a blood culture and, acting on the assumption that the cause may be bacteraemia, commence a broad spectrum antibiotic such as gentamicin or tobramycin while awaiting the result of the culture.

10. Hypertension

When the blood pressure is elevated, care is needed in giving sodium-containing solutions, which may elevate it still further. They may also produce congestive heart failure and pulmonary oedema. Hypertension may be evidence of chronic renal failure.

11. Cardiac assessment

Apart from the blood pressure it is important to assess over-all cardiac function. The importance of the elevation of the jugular venous pressure as a sign of fluid overload has been mentioned and is a sign of cardiac defeat even in the absence of overload. If this is present intravenous infusion will not be well tolerated and pulmonary oedema may develop. Intravenous infusions should be given very slowly or discontinued until the cardiac state improves.

The heart rate and rhythm are important signs. Tachycardia may be a sign of haemorrhage but may also be due to infection or to a toxic state. An ECG may be needed to decide whether it is sinus tachycardia or other arrhythmia. In some circumstances it may be useful to digitalise the patient, keeping the intravenous fluid allowance low until the full benefit of digitalis is obtained, then correcting the abnormality slowly over several days.

The auscultatory signs of importance include the presence of a pericardial rub. This may be due to a myocardial infarct, uraemic pericarditis or viral pericarditis. Uraemic pericarditis is a very rare occurrence in acute renal failure and therefore unless the patient is known or suspected to have chronic renal failure, some other explanation is more likely.

If a cardiac murmur is present and is thought to be of recent origin bacterial endocarditis should be considered and a series of blood cultures taken.

12. Lungs

Important signs may be discovered during examination of the lungs. The presence or absence of dyspnoea should be noted. Severe dyspnoea with cyanosis, associated with copious frothy, sometimes pink or blood-stained sputum is characteristic of acute pulmonary oedema. Bubbling crepitations are heard all over the chest.

Dullness on percussion, impaired or absent breath sounds and voice conduction are present with pleural effusion. Fine basal crepitations may be the first sign of fluid overload.

13. Anaemia

When anaemia is associated with hypotension blood loss must be excluded before considering other possibilities.

Anaemia that worsens over a few days, without obvious signs of blood loss, may be due to haemolysis. The haemolysis may be due to drugs or to bacterial toxins. An important and serious form of this condition, often associated with sepsis, is disseminated intravascular coagulation (synonyms: microangiopathic haemolytic anaemia, consumption coagulopathy). Besides anaemia with fragmented red cells and burr cells, thrombocytopenia is present and fibrin degradation products appear in the urine. When a very ill patient develops a progressive fall in haemoglobin and platelet count over a few days it is important to consider this diagnosis. In severe cases intractable haemorrhage from gastrointestinal tract may occur. It is treated by giving small doses of heparin, as well as treating the cause of infection.

Anaemia may have been present before the patient became ill, and normochromic, normocytic anaemia is suggestive of chronically impaired renal function.

14. Abdomen

Inspection of the abdomen may be very informative. There may be dressings saturated with bile or fluid coming from an intestinal fistula. Fluids may be collected into drainage bags, either directly or via a tube drain, without the loss being recorded on the fluid balance chart.

The abdominal wall may bear the scars of operations and their position may suggest an operation for diversion of ureters into the colon, which frequently leads to hyperchloraemic acidosis with severe hypokalaemia and often to chronic impairment of renal function.

The abdomen may be distended and percussion may indicate that this is largely due to distended loops of bowel, or to fluid free in the abdominal cavity. The absence of bowel sounds may indicate paralytic ileus, when large amounts of fluid may be effectively 'lost' into distended loops of intestine. If no bowel sounds are heard, ask the patient if flatus has been passed recently, and listen again to avoid mistaking a silent interval for paralytic ileus.

It is important to palpate the bladder area and percuss it carefully. A full bladder is a surprisingly frequent finding in a patient reported as being anuric.

15. Tendon reflexes

The knee and ankle reflexes may be reduced or absent in severe hypokalaemia. However, they may persist even with very low levels of potassium. Paresis of the lower limbs may occur with very low but also with very high potassium levels. However, paresis is a very rare sign of abnormally high plasma potassium levels – seen only three times in over 20 years of interest in electrolyte problems. An ECG is a rapid screening test for hypo- or hyperkalaemia (Chapter 15).

16. Restless patient

A full bladder is a common cause of restlessness – which may be extreme. It is important to remember that women as well as men may develop retention of urine. This is sometimes mistaken for anuria.

Restlessness may be an early sign of hypernatraemia, in contrast to the apathy and mental slowing seen in hyponatraemia.

17. Fontanelle in infancy

The state of the fontanelle is a useful sign in infancy. If retracted it suggests hypovolaemia. If protruding water and sodium overload may be present, provided intra-cranial causes can be excluded.

6. Fluid balance records and their interpretation

1. Fluid balance chart

Fluid balance charts are invaluable when used for the right patients in the right way. Keeping a fluid balance chart entails the measurement of unpleasant excreta and makes extra work for the nursing staff. Therefore, they should be used only for patients who really require them and they should be discontinued as soon as the need for them is over.

Fluid balance charts are essential for the proper treatment of the severely injured, patients who have recently undergone surgery, patients receiving intravenous fluids, and patients with impaired cardiac, renal or hepatic function during acute illness.

The fluid balance chart should record all fluid administered and excreted. Each route of intake and excretion should be recorded in a separate column and care should be taken that the entries are legible and entered in the correct column. All fluids should be measured in millilitres. The chart should be used on one side only for intake and output records and should be sufficiently large to cover a period of 24 hours. It is essential to date each chart. It may be convenient to use the reverse side of the sheet for the recording of the daily prescription for intravenous fluids, recording the time for commencing and completing each container of fluid.

The chart used in the Belfast City Hospital is shown in Figs. 7 and 8. It will be noted that the chart commences at 10.00 hours. This is a convenient time to order the daily fluid intake, which is based on the previous day's output. In many hospitals the chart commences at 08.00 hours, a time when medical staff are not usually in the ward. The duty nurse then has to decide between telephoning the doctor for a prescription for the next fluid to be given, slowing down the existing drip to make the fluid last until he arrives, or putting up a new bottle on her own initiative.

The chart ends with a tear-off slip, gummed on the reverse side, which contains a summary of intake and output for a 24-hour period, with a space for recording the date. This slip can become part of the permanent chart without greatly increasing the bulk of the chart. The nurse should never discard the complete record until it has been verified by the doctor. It is useful to retain at least the previous two days' charts in case any query arises and in really ill patients it is advisable to retain the complete records until the patient recovers.

There are drawbacks to the Belfast chart in use and this is probably true of all charts yet devised. Some still prefer a chart running from 08.00 to 08.00 hours. It is

DAILY FLUID CHART				AFFIX LABEL HERE OR ENTER				
24 Hours Beginning				FULL NAME				
				HOSPITAL NUMBER				
				CONSULTANT				

	INTAKE				OUTPUT				REMARKS
TIME	Intake by Mouth		Intravenous or other routes		Urine	Faeces	Vomit	Tube	
	Amount	Type	Amount	Type					
1000 hrs									
1100 hrs									
1200 hrs									
1300 hrs									
1400 hrs									
1500 hrs									
1600 hrs									
1700 hrs									
1800 hrs									
1900 hrs									
2000 hrs									
2100 hrs									
2200 hrs.									
2300 hrs.									
2400 hrs.									
0100 hrs.									
0200 hrs									
0300 hrs									
0400 hrs.									
0500 hrs.									
0600 hrs.									
0700 hrs									
0800 hrs									
0900 hrs.									

	INTAKE			OUTPUT				
Day Total	By Mouth	Intravenous or other routes	Urine	Faeces	Vomit	Tube	Date
	ML	ML	ML		ML	ML	
Night Total	ML	ML	ML		ML	ML	
Total for 24 hrs	ML	ML	ML		ML	ML	
TOTAL INTAKE			TOTAL OUTPUT				

Fig. 7. Fluid chart in use in Belfast City Hospital.

easier to use a chart with which everyone is familiar and it is best if one pattern of chart is used throughout the hospital so that all staff become familiar with the chart and its usage.

The chart should be checked daily by the doctor and it should be made clear to the nursing staff that it is used as a basis for the intravenous fluid prescription.

		PARTICULARS OF INTRAVENOUS FLUIDS TO BE TAKEN				
Bottle	Amount	Type of Fluid	Time to be commenced	Time completed	Initials	
1						
2						
3						
4						
5						

1 litre 0 9% Na Cl ("normal saline") contains 155 m Eq. Na and 155 m Eq Cl
1 litre M/6 Na lactate contains 162 m Eq Na and 162 m Eq lactate (The lactate is converted to bicarbonate in the body)
1 g Na Cl contains 17 25 m Eq Na and 17 25 m Eq Cl
1 g Na H$_2$CO$_3$ contains 11 9 m Eq Na and 11 9 m Eq H$_2$CO$_3$.
1 g K Cl contains 13 5 m Eq K and 13 5 m Eq Cl
1 g K citrate contains 9 3 m Eq K and 9 3 m Eq citrate
1 g Na lactate contains 9 0 m Eq Na and 9 0 m Eq lactate

N.B. Patients receiving intravenous therapy only for periods of longer than 48 hours require potassium replacement as well as sodium replacement if there is any sizeable loss of intestinal contents, even if oliguric. They may be oliguric because of potassium deficiency If in doubt ask for expert advice

N.B. It is dangerous to correct "acidosis" on the basis of the "base deficit" on the Astrup estimation without knowledge of the plasma Na value It is permissible for the expert to do this in emergency situations such as cardiac arrest

DO NOT PRESCRIBE INTRAVENOUS FLUIDS WITHOUT FIRST CONSIDERING PREVIOUS OUTPUT, WHETHER CHARTERED OR ESTIMATED FROM HISTORY

Fig. 8. Fluid record chart in use in Belfast City Hospital. Reverse is used for prescription of intravenous fluids

The attention of the nurse in charge should be drawn to any entries which are not clearly marked in the proper columns. The arithmetic should always be checked.

2. Fluid intake

There should be separate columns for the recording of oral and intravenous fluids. The volume of semi-solid foods taken should be recorded also.

Sources of confusion may arise from the method of recording. The full volume of a jug of water or other beverage is sometimes recorded when it is left on the locker, regardless of the fact that much of the fluid may still remain in the jug when it is taken away again. Ideally fluid should be recorded on the chart at the time it is actually taken, but this is often impossible to achieve in a busy ward. Similarly the total amount contained in the intravenous bottle or container is sometimes recorded at the time it is commenced, but the drip may stop and part of the fluid be discarded when a new intravenous infusion is commenced. It is better to record the volume given at the time when administration is completed. An even more confusing practice is that of recording the diminishing volume in the container at regular intervals, which may make it appear to the uninitiated that vast quantities of fluid had been given. This practice seems to be common in paediatric wards, and is supposed to guard against too rapid administration of the day's prescribed intravenous fluids.

2.1. Unrecorded sources of fluid intake

There may be unrecorded sources of fluid intake some of which are listed in Table 12.

Table 12. Unrecorded sources of fluid intake.

1. Central venous mamometer
2. Arterial cannula
3. 'Piggy-back' drip
4. Correction of acidosis
5. Aludrox
6. Water content of humidified air or steam tent

2.1.1. Central venous manometer
The central venous manometer if properly used, does not require the infusion of fluid into the patient. However, the tap may be maladjusted, or left turned on while the doctor's attention is distracted from the measurement he is making, and a considerable amount of saline infused. The central venous manometer should be needed for only a short period at the beginning of the illness or in theatre, and should be dispensed with as soon as possible.

2.1.2. Arterial cannula
In intensive care units, where frequent sampling of arterial blood is needed to check the adequacy of ventilation, it is customary to insert an arterial cannula which requires to be flushed at regular intervals to keep it patent. About 40 ml of saline per 24 hours ought to be sufficient for this purpose, but on occasion much more is used, and is not recorded.

2.1.3. Piggy-back drip
Some antibiotics must be given intravenously in dilute solution. These are often given by a 'piggy-back' drip inserted into the main intravenous line. The volume of this extra fluid is sometimes overlooked.

2.1.4. Correction of acidosis

Sodium bicarbonate solution may be given on the result of the arterial sample. When ventilation is inadequate, carbon dioxide is retained leading to respiratory acidosis. The reason why this should not be done has been described already in Chapter 3.

2.1.5. Aludrox

In severely ill patients Aludrox is given via the intragastric tube for prophylaxis against acute peptic ulceration. In the usual dose of 30 ml at 2-hour intervals, this amounts to 360 ml per 24 hours.

2.1.6. Water content of humidified gases or steam tent

When a patient is ventilated with humidified gasses loss of water by respiration ceases. The usual 500 ml of water allowed for insensible loss should be reduced to 200 ml.

3. Fluid output

There should be separate columns for the recording of urine, vomitus or aspiration, faecal loss, loss from drainage tubes or fistula. In most wards the urinary and gastric losses are measured and recorded, but faecal loss is seldom measured.

3.1. Unrecorded fluid losses

Occasionally the patient has a considerable faecal loss, even to the extent of frequent diarrhoeal motions, without it being recorded on the chart at all, probably because it is a more unpleasant task to measure faeces than urine or even vomitus. Vomiting is often a sudden event occurring over the bed-clothes rather than into a basin, and no measurement is possible. Losses from fistula or drains into dressings are often not recorded. Moreover, the busy nurse who goes to the sluice to measure the fluid loss, whatever it is, may be diverted to some other task before she has recorded the event on the chart. Loss due to excessive sweating is unlikely to be mentioned. Therefore, the losses recorded on the chart should be regarded as minimal losses and a search made for other possible sources of loss.

4. Prescription for intravenous fluids

The prescription for intravenous fluids, after any initial deficit is replaced, is based on the fluid loss over the preceding 24 hours, plus an allowance to cover insensible loss through the skin and respiration. It is much safer to prescribe on the basis of the

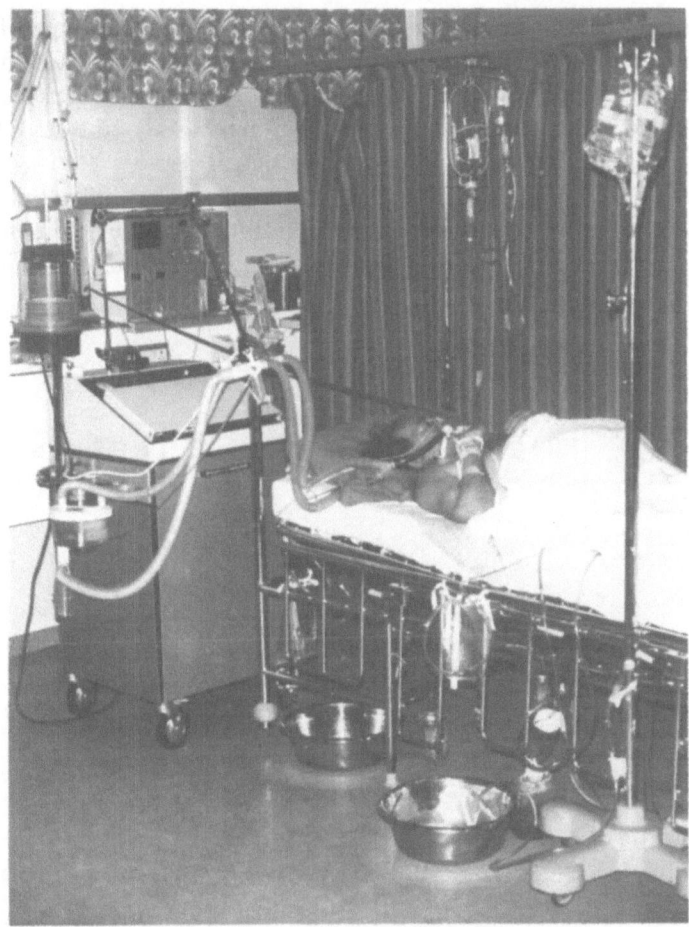

Fig. 9. The difficulties encountered in accurately assessing fluid intake and output in patients receiving intensive care are shown by this patient on a respirator who is receiving humidified gases, has a nasogastric tube and urethral catheter, is receiving parenteral fluids and an antibiotic by a piggy-back infusion line, and who requires peritoneal dialysis.

previous day's output than to anticipate the possible loss over the current 24 hours. Even if the loss by urine and other routes increases considerably, in one 24-hour period it is unlikely that the patient will become seriously depleted. A possible exception to this rule is the period immediately following relief of urinary obstruction when very large amounts of dilute urine may be passed. In these circumstances it is advisable to check the output every 12 hours and prescribe accordingly. If the prescription were to be based on anticipated output, the loss might, in fact, be very much less than expected, for example, because of a fall in blood pressure, and the patient might become fluid overloaded. Slight dehydration is preferable to fluid overload with its attendant risks of congestive heart failure, and pulmonary oedema.

The fluids to be given should be clearly recorded on the reverse of the fluid balance chart, or other chart designed for this purpose. The volume, type of fluid and concentration, the time for commencing and finishing each container of fluid should be recorded and the prescription signed by the doctor who prescribes it. It may sometimes be necessary to change the prescription because of the day's laboratory results, and if a change is made this should be signed also.

The accurate recording of fluid intake and output can be difficult in patients in intensive care units, who may be on a respiratory breathing humidified gases, receiving parenteral nutrition, drugs through a piggy-back infusion line and require peritoneal dialysis (Fig. 9).

7. Laboratory data and useful investigations

1. Chemical substances in body fluids

It should be remembered that in clinical laboratories because of the large workload it is usual to measure the concentration of chemical substances once only on each specimen. The precision attained is therefore well below that considered acceptable in academic laboratories, where specimens are usually measured in duplicate or triplicate and the mean used as the true value. Individual laboratories vary somewhat in their range of reference values and it is important to know the reference ranges of the laboratory with which one works. This has become even more important with the change to SI units as for many chemicals the numerical range has been considerably reduced, thus increasing the significance of small inter-laboratory differences.

Some chemical substances are more difficult to measure accurately than others. Two which present special difficulty because of dietary influence or interference from other substances are calcium and creatinine. An unexpectedly high or low value for either requires to be checked on a second specimen of blood.

When automated methods of analysis are used, specimens are estimated in batches. The precision (in terms of coefficient of variation) of most laboratory estimations is least good in the lower range of the calibration curve. When the actual concentration in a specimen is outside the analytical range of the method, the sample should be diluted (2-, 5- or 10-fold as appropriate) and the estimation repeated. The technician in the laboratory is often unaware that a very high level is expected and the whole batch has been completed before the high value is noted, a dilution made, and the test repeated. This leads to delay in reporting the abnormal result to the ward. When writing the request form the doctor can help by indicating that an abnormally high value may be present, if he suspects this to be the case.

2. Chemical substances in serum/plasma

The reference range for chemical substances other than enzymes and hormones in serum/plasma is given in Table 13. When obtaining the blood specimen care should be taken to avoid haemolysis, which is particularly likely to occur if there are bubbles present. Haemolysis produces a misleadingly high level for potassium and phosphate. Blood specimens should be withdrawn without undue stasis which may

Table 13. Reference range for chemical substances in serum/plasma.

	Constituent	SI units		Former units			Conversion factors SI to former units
		Reference range	Units	Reference range		Units	multiply by
S	Albumen	36 – 53	g/l	3.5 – 5.3		g/100 ml	0.1
P	Bicarbonate	20 – 30	mmol/l	20 – 30		mEq/l	1
S	Bilirubin (total)	3 – 17	μmol/l	0.2 – 1.0		mg/100 ml	0.0585
S	Calcium	2.30 – 2.62	mmol/l	9.2 – 10.5		mg/100 ml	4.008
P	Chloride	99 – 108	mmol/l	99 – 108		mg/100 ml	1
S	Cholesterol	2.8 – 9.8	mmol/l	110 – 380		mg/100 ml	38.7
S	Creatinine	55 – 120	μmol/l	0.6 – 1.4		mg/100 ml	0.011
S	Complement C_3	0.45 – 1.00	g/l	–		–	–
S	Complement C_4	0.18 – 0.42	g/l	–		–	–
S	C-reactive protein	0 – 0.06	g/l	–		–	–
S	Copper	13.0 – 27.0	μmol/l	83 – 171		μg/100 ml	6.35
S	Ferritin						
	females	10 – 75	μg/l	–		–	–
	males	12 – 200	μg/l	–		–	–
P	Fibrinogen	2 – 4	g/l	200 – 400		mg/100 ml	100
S	Folate	1.5 – 5.5	μg/l	–		–	–
S	Globulin	18 – 36	g/l	1.8 – 3.6		g/100 ml	0.1
P	Glucose (fasting)	3.3 – 5.5	mmol/l	60 – 100		mg/100 ml	18.02
S	Immunoglobulins						
	IgG	6.50 – 16.0	g/l	650 – 1600		mg/100 ml	100
	IgA	1.00 – 4.50	g/l	100 – 450		mg/100 ml	100
	IgM	0.45 – 2.00	g/l	45 – 200		mg/100 ml	100
S	Iron	7.0 – 45.0	μmol/l	40 – 250		μg/100 ml	5.59
S	Total iron-binding capacity	45.0 – 73.0	μmol/l	250 – 410		μg/100 ml	5.59
B	Lactate	0.7 – 1.8	mmol/l	6.0 – 16.0		mg/100 ml	9
S	Lipids						
	cholesterol	2.8 – 9.8	mmol/l	110 – 380		mg/100 ml	38.7
	triglycerides	0.30 – 1.50	mmol/l	26 – 130		mg/100 ml	88.5
S	Magnesium	0.80 – 1.07	mmol/l	1.9 – 2.6		mg/100 ml	2.43
P	Osmolality	280 – 300	mmol/kg	280 – 300		mosmol/kg	1
S	Phosphate (as inorganic P)	0.6 – 1.5	mmol/l[↓]	2.0 – 4.5[↓]		mg/100 ml	3.10
P	Potassium	3.8 – 4.8	mmol/l	3.8 – 4.8		mEq/l	1
P	Protein						
	total	63 – 79	g/l	6.3 – 7.9		g/100 ml	0.1
	albumen	36 – 53	g/l	3.6 – 5.3		g/100 ml	0.1
	globulin	18 – 36	g/l	1.8 – 3.6		g/100 ml	0.1
B	Pyruvate	40 – 80	μmol/l	0.36 – 0.72		mg/100 ml	0.009
P	Sodium	135 – 145	mmol/l	135 – 145		mEq/l	1
P	Urea	3.3 – 6.7	mmol/l	20 – 40		mg/100 ml	6.01
P	Urate	170 – 500	μmol/l	2.8 – 8.4		mg/100 ml	0.017
S	Zinc	7.7 – 23.0	μmol/l	50 – 150		μg/100 ml	6.537

[↓] = Higher levels for children.

cause artefactual elevation of some constituents especially calcium and protein. It is permissible whilst entering the vein to use a tourniquet, which is released before withdrawing the blood sample.

The serum calcium exists partly as protein-bound calcium (about 40%) partly as ionized calcium (about 50–56%) and the remainder as non-protein-bound ultrafilterable calcium complexed to citrate. The ionized calcium is important for calcium homeostasis, bone metabolism, nerve conduction and blood clotting. It has been technically very difficult to measure ionized calcium until recently and although simpler methods using the calcium electrode are now available the equipment is expensive.

Total serum calcium only is measured in most hospital laboratories and is quite satisfactory for most clinical purposes. Some authorities insist that the serum calcium must be measured in the fasting state but I have not found this to be important. It is useful, however, to measure the plasma protein concentration in the same specimen of blood. Any deviation from normal of the plasma proteins requires a correction to the measured total calcium concentration, but there is no generally accepted rule for the correction. Dr Alan Rose suggests that a reference value for total plasma protein be taken as 70 g/l and for each change in plasma protein of 10 g/l the total serum calcium should be corrected by 0.188 mmol/l. Where the total serum protein is less than the reference value, the correction should be added to the measured serum calcium concentration and where the total serum protein is greater than the reference value, the correction should be subtracted.

The serum phosphate concentration is higher in infancy and childhood than in adults. This is important when considering a diagnosis of familial hypophosphataemic rickets.

It is sometimes useful to compare the serum concentrations of urea and creatinine. The urea concentration reflects the nitrogen present in the protein of the diet as well as renal function. Occasionally the chance observation of a raised urea concentration in the absence of other indications of impaired renal function may cause concern. This is sometimes due to consumption of a very high protein, low carbohydrate diet for slimming purposes, when the serum creatinine concentration and the creatinine clearance remain normal. Bleeding into the upper gastrointestinal tract has a similar effect, leading to elevation of the serum urea out of proportion to the serum creatinine. Very low protein high carbohydrate diets prescribed for patients with advanced renal failure and not yet on dialysis have the opposite effect – a reduction of the serum urea concentration despite continued elevation of the serum creatinine.

The plasma protein concentration, when measured serially in the same patient, can be used to monitor changes in hydration.

Table 14. Reference range for enzymes and hormones in serum/plasma.

	Constituent	SI units		Former units		Conversion SI to former units multiply by
		Reference range	Units	Reference range	Units	
P	ACTH	10 – 70	ng/l	10 – 70	u/l	1
S	Aspartate transaminase (AST)	2 – 35	IU/l	2 – 35	u/l	1
P	Alanine transaminase (ALT)	7 – 45	IU/l	1 – 12	IU/l	*
S	Aldolase	0.5 – 3.1	U/l			1
S	Amylase	70 – 300	U/l	75 – 200	Somogyi/100 ml	*
P	Catecholamines (as noradrenaline)	Less than 11	nmol/l	less than 2	µg/l	0.169
S	Cholinesterase ('pseudocholinesterase')	3.0 – 9.3	U/l			
S	Caeruloplasmin	0.27 – 0.63	g/l	27 – 63	mg/100 ml	100
P	Cortisol evening	Less than 150	nmol/l	less than 5	µg/100 ml	0.036
	morning	150 – 700		5 – 25	µg/100 ml	
P	Creatine kinase (CK)	10 – 120	U/l			*
P	Gamma-glutamyltransferase (GGT)	5 – 60	U/l	4 – 28	U/l	*
S	Gastrin	up to 100	ng/l			
S	Glucagon N-terminal	up to 250	ng/l			
S	C-terminal	up to 150	ng/l			
S	Haptoglobin	0.35 – 2.50 as Hb-binding capacity	g/l			
	Growth hormone		S			0 – 1.0 µg/l
S	Hydroxybutyrate dehydrogenase	55 – 140	U/l	55 – 140	U/l	1
S	Insulin	5 – 15	mU/l			
S	Lactate dehydrogenase (LD)	240 – 440	U/l			
B	Luteinising hormone (LH) males	0.4 – 6.0	U/l			
	females	0.4 – 12.0	U/l			

Table 14. Continued.

Constituent	SI units		Former units		Conversion SI to former units multiply by
	Reference range	Units	Reference range	Units	
P Oestradiol					
males	22 – 160	pmol/l			
females					
follicular phase	73 – 460	pmol/l			
luteal phase	165 – 700	pmol/l			
ovulatory peak	280 – 1250	pmol/l			
P Parathyroid hormone (PTH)	0.3 – 0.7	µg/l			
S Phosphatase acid (ACP) (tartrate-labile)	0.0 – 2.0	U/l	0 – 0.8	KA U/100 ml	*
S Phosphatase alkaline (ALP) adult	50 – 170	U/l‡	3 – 14	KA U/100 ml	*
B Progesterone					
males	0.16 – 1.29	nmol/l			
females					
follicular phase	0.16 – 1.9	nmol/l			
luteal phase	6.3 – 80	nmol/l			
luteal peak	greater than 30	nmol/l			
S Secretin	up to 50	ng/l			
P Testosterone					
males	9.4 – 24.3	nmol/l			
females	0.7 – 2.4	nmol/l			
P Thyroid stimulating hormone (TSH)					
males	1.5 – 7.2	mU/l			
females	1.5 – 5.5	mU/l			
P Thyroxine (T$_4$)	70 – 160	nmol/l	5.4 – 12.4	µg/100 ml	0.078
P Triiodothyronine (T$_3$)	1.2 – 2.8	nmol/l	0.8 – 1.8	ng/ml	0.65

* = Direct conversion not possible.
‡ = Higher values in children.

3. Enzymes and hormones in serum/plasma

The reference values for the enzymes and hormones usually measured in hospital laboratories are given in Table 14.

The methods for estimation of hormones are often very complicated and an error at any stage will produce a misleading value. For certain hormones, including parathyroid hormone (PTH), gastrin and other intestinal hormones, the hormone rapidly disappears in blood left at room temperature. The tube containing the specimen must be put into ice chips as quickly as possible and taken at once to the laboratory where it must be centrifuged in a refrigerated centrifuge. Gastrin and other gastrointestinal hormones should be measured after the patient has fasted overnight.

4. Acid/base and gaseous components of blood

When it is desired to measure pH and gaseous components of blood, it is essential to obtain the specimen free from air bubbles. Arterial blood is usually used, but capillary blood obtained without statis may be used if there is no evidence of circulatory failure.

pH, P_{CO_2} and P_{O_2} are measured by specific electrodes [3]. P_{CO_2} may be measured also by the equilibration method of Astrup [1] but modern pH and blood gas analysers now use the specific electrode technique.

Instrument problems are common and the oxygen electrode may sometimes give reproducible and stable readings which are 'clinically crazy'. It is useful as a safeguard against instrument failure to always observe the colour of the blood in the syringe. The P_{O_2} of pink blood is above 50 mm Hg, when cyanosis can just be detected the P_{O_2} is about 40 mm Hg, and when the blood is blue-black the P_{O_2} in less than 30 mm Hg.

5. Base excess and buffer base

In clinical practice it is much easier to plan treatment on the basis of a measurement expressed in mmol/l rather than on the pH value [2]. Siggaard-Andersen and Engel provided two scales on their original nomogram enabling both base excess and buffer base in mmol/l to be read off. *Base excess* gives in mmol/l the amount of *acid* required to restore the pH of a blood sample to normal, at body temperature (37°C) and normal P_{CO_2} (40 mm Hg) while *base deficit* gives in mmol/l the amount of *base* required to restore pH to normal under the same conditions. *Buffer base* is the sum of the anions bicarbonate and protein and therefore depends upon the haemoglobin concentration of whole blood. The parameters base excess and buffer base may be provided, using an algorithm, as part of the results display on modern pH and blood gas analysers.

6. Actual and standard bicarbonate

The actual bicarbonate concentration is the total available bicarbonate buffer provided by both the erythrocyte and renal mechanisms. It is calculated from the Henderson-Hasselbalch equation using the measured pH and Pco_2 values.

The standard bicarbonate concentration is the amount of bicarbonate buffer which would be present if the Pco_2 of the blood were at a standard value of 40 mm Hg.

In acute respiratory disturbance, for example, the difference between the actual bicarbonate and the standard bicarbonate represents the contribution made to the bicarbonate buffer concentration by the erythrocytes.

The standard bicarbonate is calculated from the Henderson-Hasselbalch equation using the measured pH and a Pco_2 of 40 mm Hg. As for base excess and buffer base, the actual and standard bicarbonate concentrations may be displayed as part of the results profile on a blood gas analyser.

7. Plasma total CO_2 (TCO_2), plasma bicarbonate

This is normally measured as part of the electrolyte block and is a measure of the sum of the plasma concentrations of bicarbonate, carbonic acid and dissolved CO_2. Since only 1 mmol/l and between 1 and 2 mmol/l is contributed by carbonic acid and dissolved CO_2 respectively, the total CO_2 is effectively a measure of plasma bicarbonate concentration.

The reference values for arterial blood pH, Pco_2, and Po_2, total bicarbonate, standard bicarbonate and base excess are given in Table 15.

Information about the Pco_2 is valuable in two ways. If the measured value is close to the normal value of 40 mm Hg (Range 38–42) then any change in pH from normal must be metabolic rather than respiratory in origin. On the other hand if the measured value for Pco_2 is abnormal it may be an indication of respiratory acidosis or alkalosis as the case may be.

An elevation of the Pco_2 is present in respiratory acidosis and a reduction of the Pco_2 is present in respiratory alkalosis. In respiratory disturbances the primary event is either failure of removal of CO_2 (acidosis from an excess of H^+ ions in H_2CO_3) or excessive loss of CO_2 (alkalosis from a reduction in the proportion of H_2CO_3). It should be noted that Pco_2 is used to assess the respiratory component and CO_2 from the electrolyte block the metabolic component of acid/base abnormality.

Blood pH and blood gas values may be very helpful during first assessment of a

Table 15. Blood acid base and blood gas values.

	SI units		Former units		Conversion SI to former units
	Reference range	Units	Reference range	Units	multiply by
Hydrogen ion concentration	36 – 45	nmol/l	pH 7.35 – pH 7.44		–
P_{CO_2}	4.7 – 6.0	kPa	35.0 – 45.0 mm Hg		7.52
P_{O_2}	12.0 – 14.6	kPa	90.0 – 110.0 mm Hg		7.52
Total CO_2	24.0 – 30.0	mmol/l	24.0 – 30.0 mEq/l		1
Standard bicarbonate	22.0 – 26.0	mmol/l	22.0 – 26.0 mEq/l		1
Base excess	±2.5	mmol/l	±2.5	mEq/l	1

patient with electrolyte disturbance but are usually *not* required for day-to-day management of intravenous therapy. The electrolyte block contains the basic biochemical information needed for daily prescription of intravenous fluids. However, daily or frequent blood pH and blood gas values are essential for the management of patients with respiratory problems on respirators.

In all circumstances the results of the biochemical tests must be considered along with the clinical history and the findings on physical examination.

8. Chemical substances in urine

The reference range for the urinary excretion of chemical substances other than hormones and enzymes is given in Table 16. A little toluene is added to the urine container to act as a preservative, except for the specimen to be used for measurement of urinary calcium excretion, when acetic acid is added to the container to prevent precipitation of calcium salts.

A 24-hour collection of urine is required for these tests, and it is important that the collection should be complete. It can be surprisingly difficult to obtain complete urine collections in general hospital wards, mainly because of frequent changes of duty nurses. It is usually best to explain the test to the patient, as well as to the duty nurse, and to make the patient responsible for ensuring that no urine samples are discarded. Most patients can collect satisfactory 24-hour specimens at home provided that the details of the test are explained clearly, backed up with written instructions, and a 2-litre container is provided (Appendix 2).

Measurement of the 24-hour excretion of urinary electrolytes is helpful in acute renal failure (especially in 'high output' failure) and in chronic renal failure.

In acutely ill patients and following severe trauma it is very useful to monitor the hourly urinary output by a urinometer attached to the urethral catheter. A urinary

Table 16. Reference range for chemical substances excreted in urine.

Constituent	SI units		Former units		Conversion SI to former units
	Reference range	Units/24 hr	Reference range	Units/24 hr	multiply by
Calcium	2.5 – 7.5	mmol	0.1 – 0.3	g	0.04
Chloride	100 – 250	mmol	100 – 250	mEq	1
Copper	0.2 – 1.6	µmol	13 – 102	µg	63.5
Creatinine	9 – 18	mmol	1 – 2	g	0.113
Creatinine clearance	90 – 120	ml/min			
Cystine	less than 125	µmol	less than 30	mg	0.24
Hydroxyproline[a]					
0– 1 yr	420 – 1680	$\mu mol.m^{-2}$	55 – 220	$mg.m^{-2}$	
1–13 yr	190 – 610	$\mu mol.m^{-2}$	25 – 80	$mg.m^{-2}$	0.1311
22–65 yr	46 – 168	$\mu mol.m^{-2}$	6 – 22	$mg.m^{-2}$	
over 65 yr	38 – 160	$\mu mol.m^{-2}$	5 – 21	$mg.m^{-2}$	
Lead	0 – 0.40	µmol	0 – 83	µg	207
Osmolality[b]	15 – 1300	mmol/kg	15 – 1300	mosmol/kg	1
					Phosphate
(as inorganic P)	15 – 50	mmol	0.5 – 1.5	g	0.031
Potassium	25 – 100	mmol	25 – 100	mEq	1
Protein (total)	less than 0.200	g	less than 0.200	g	1
Sodium	120 – 220	mmol	120 – 220	mEq	1
Urate	1.5 – 4.5	mmol	0.25 – 0.75	g	0.17
Urea	216 – 600	mmol	13 – 36	g	0.06

[a] Test to be carried out while patient is on special gelatine-free diet.
[b] Urinary osmolality is expressed as mmol/kg or mosmol/kg.

output of 50 ml/hr or more is good evidence that perfusion of the kidneys is adequate.

9. Enzymes and hormones in urine

The reference range for the urinary excretion of some enzymes and hormones is given in Table 17. A 24-hour urine collection is required for these tests. For some tests special precautions are needed in the collection of urine, or the laboratory needs advance information to prepare reagents, etc. It is, therefore, advisable to consult your own laboratory before arranging for the 24-hour collection of urine.

Table 17. Reference range for enzymes and hormones excreted in urine.

Constituent	SI units		Former units		Conversion SI to former units
	Reference range	Units/24 hr	Reference range	Units/24 hr	multiply by
Amylase	100 – 2000	U	–		–
Catecholamines					
(as noradrenaline)	less than 0.65	μmol	less than 110	μg	169
Cortisol					
adult males	300 – 1090	nmol	109 – 395	μg	0.3625
adult females	205 – 845	nmol	74 – 306	μg	0.3625
FSH					
children	0.7 – 2	U	0.7 – 2	U	1
females					
pre-and post-					
ovulation	2 – 10	U	2 – 10	U	1
ovulatory	8 – 26	U	8 – 26	U	
postmenopausal	10 – 65	U	10 – 65	U	
males	2 – 12	U	2 – 12	U	1
5-hydroxyindole					
acetate (5HIAA)	10 – 42	μmol	1.9 – 8.0	mg	0.19
4-hydroxy 3-methoxy					
mandelate (VMA)	5 – 38	μmol	1.0 – 7.6	mg	0.2
Luteinising hormone					
children	2.5 – 10	U			
females					
pre- and post-					
ovulation	8 – 50	U			
ovulatory	50 – 200	U			
postmenopausal	25 – 180	U			
males	9 – 40	U			

10. Renal function tests

10.1. Serum urea

The measurement of serum urea is a readily available routine test. However, results can be misleading, as an elevated serum urea concentration does not always indicate impaired renal function, either acute or chronic, e.g., a high protein low calorie diet increases the serum urea concentration. Similarly, when a protein restricted diet is used for treatment of chronic renal failure, the urea is misleadingly low.

10.2. Serum creatinine

An elevation of serum creatinine concentration is usually significant, the concentration depending to some extent on muscle mass as well as on renal function.

10.3. Creatinine clearance

Creatinine clearance gives an approximate measurement of glomerular filtration rate. However, at low levels of renal function it is an overestimate because creatinine is secreted by tubules as well as filtered at glomerulus. It requires a 24-hour collection of urine accompanied by 5 ml clotted blood. It is a non-invasive test which is easily carried out and can be repeated as frequently as needed on outpatients. Fairly reproducible values are obtained when the patient is responsible for collection of his own urine. Serial values are very useful for monitoring renal function.

A disadvantage is the need for a *complete* 24-hour urine collection. Calculation:

$$\frac{\text{Creatinine}}{\text{clearance}} = \frac{\text{Urine volume (ml/min)} \times \text{urine concentration } (\mu\text{mol/l})}{\text{serum concentration } (\mu\text{mol/l})} \text{ ml/min}$$

Metabolic rates are in general related to body size. The observed clearance rate can be corrected to motional normal adult body surface area (SA) of 1.73 m² from height and weight from the nomogram of Sendroy and Cecchini [4] from the formula of Dubois and Dubois [5]

$$SA = \text{height}^{0.725} \times \text{weight}^{0.425} \times 71.84$$

10.4. Inulin clearance

This gives a more accurate measurement of glomerular filtration rate than creatinine clearance but requires constant intravenous infusion of inulin and very accurate urine collection (but a short period is sufficient). It is not suitable for regular clinical use but is used in renal physiology. With good renal function, values for inulin clearance follow closely those obtained by simultaneous measurement of creatinine clearance (the tubular secretion of creatinine is offset by the method of estimation of serum creatinine which also measures other substances present in serum to give a slightly high serum value).

10.5. Clearance using radioactive substances

This method requires intravenous injection of either chromium-labelled EDTA or radioactive-labelled vitamin B_{12} and facilities for their subsequent measurement in serum and urine. This method provides a more accurate measurement of glomerular filtration rate than does creatinine clearance especially at low levels of function.

10.6. Urinary protein

Urinary protein excretion is measured in a 24-hour collection of urine. The reference range for adults is less than 200 mg/24 hours, but vaginal discharge and menstruation may give falsely high levels in females.

10.7. Urine concentration tests

These are seldom needed in practice and should *never* be used in patients who have impaired glomerular filtration as the dehydration required may cause acute worsening of renal function. They are of value in establishing diabetes insipidus.

The patient is instructed to abstain from fluids from 12 noon the previous day. The early morning urine should have a specific gravity of 1.022 or more.

A more precise estimate of urine-concentrating ability is given by measurement of the urine osmolality which should be greater than 850 milliosmols. A shorter period (6.00 pm to 7.00 am) of fluid and food restriction may also be used. If an inability to concentrate the urine has been established by the water deprivation test, the injection of 5 units of pitressin tannate and a repeat of the test will distinguish between pituitary and nephrogenic diabetes insipidus: there is no improvement if failure to concentrate is due to tubular disease.

10.8. Ability to acidify urine

This test is used to confirm diagnosis of renal tubular acidosis. The test is carried out by giving an oral dose of 8 g of ammonium chloride at 8.00 am. Urine samples are collected for estimation of pH at hourly intervals. With normal tubular function the resultant acidosis should lead to a fall in urinary pH to 5.2 or lower.

10.9. Selectivity of proteinuria

This gives a measure of the molecular size of protein excreted in the urine. When only small-size protein is present in the urine the proteinuria is said to be highly selective. The clearances of a small protein, such as albumen or transferrin, and a large protein, such as IgG, are measured and expressed as a ratio.

A highly selective proteinuria is indicated by a large protein to small protein clearance ratio of less than 0.2.

Highly selective proteinuria is characteristic of minimal change glomerulonephritis (but also occurs in renal diseases not primarily affecting the glomerulus). It is a useful test in childhood nephrotic syndrome, where the lesion is usually minimal change disease and the finding of highly selective proteinuria may be regarded as diagnostic, often avoiding the need for a renal biopsy. It has little value in adult renal disease, where minimal change disease is uncommon.

11. Haematological tests

The reference values for haematological tests are given in Table 18.

Table 18. Reference values for haematological tests.

Test	Male			Female			Children
RBC × 10²/l	5.5	±	1.0	4.8	±	1.0	varies with age
Hgb g/dl	15.5	±	2.5	14.0	±	2.5	average 12.5
Hct	0.47	±	0.07	0.42	±	0.05	varies with age
WBC × 10⁹/l	7.5	±	3.5	7.5	±	3.5[a]	varies with age
MCH pg	29.5	±	2.5	29.5	±	2.5	varies with age
MCV fl	85	±	8	85	±	8	varies with age
MCHC g/dl	33	±	2	33	±	2	33 ± 2
Platelets × 10⁹/l	150	–	400	150	–	400	
RDW %	9.9	±	1.4	9.9	±	1.4	
Pct %	0.224	±	0.078	0.224	±	0.078	
PCV fl	8.0	±	1.7	8.0	±	1.7	
PDW %	10	±	0.8	10	±	0.8	

[a]   Often higher in pregnancy.
fl   = femtolitres (10^{-9}).
RDW = red cell distribution width.
Pct   = platelet crit.
MPV = mean platelet volume.
PDW = platelet distribution width.

Serial measurements of the haemoglobin concentration or haematocrit can be used to monitor changes in hydration, provided that changes due to blood loss, haemolysis or transfusion can be excluded.

12. Central venous pressure (CVP)

Measurement of the central venous pressure is an invaluable aid when rapid transfusion is required, particularly during the first 24 hours after severe trauma [6].

The CVP gives information about cardiac function as well as volume. The veins and venules contain the body's reservoir of blood. A fall in this volume is partly compensated by an increase in venous tone, and partly by the pumping function of the left ventricle. A patient with a failing left ventricle needs a raised CVP to maintain normal end diastolic pressure.

The CVP is a measure of end diastolic right ventricular pressure. Right and left end diastolic pressures are usually similar and changes occur in similar direction. If the CVP is low, the left ventricular end diastolic pressure is assumed to be low, and an increase in CVP is assumed to be followed by in increase in left ventricular end pressure. The presence of lung disease (which affects the right ventricle) or ischaemic heart disease (which affects primarily the left ventricle) disturbs these normal relationships and the CVP no longer reflects left ventricular function.

The insertion of a central venous catheter is a simple procedure but it is preferable to see it carried out by an experienced operator and to do it a few times under supervision before undertaking it 'solo'. An Abbot 'drum' or other similar catheter is usually inserted via the median cubital vein into the great veins of the thorax, but the external or internal jugular veins can also be used. The patient is placed in the head down position, preferably conscious, so that the external jugular becomes distended when it is easily catheterised. Sometimes it may not be possible to pass a catheter via the external jugular because of anatomical variation from the usual configuration, and the internal jugular vein is used. The catheter in a jugular vein must be stitched in place to allow some mobility. The central venous manometer is attached to the catheter and the zero standardised to the mid-axillary line in the supine position, which approximates to the mid right atrium. The CVP is usually maintained at 8–12 cm H_2O.

13. Haemodynamic monitoring using the Swan Ganz catheter

The Swan Ganz catheter is used for haemodynamic monitoring in seriously ill patients, especially when cardiac defeat is present or suspected.

The Swan Ganz catheter has an inflatable balloon near its tip which allows it to be inserted through the right atrium and right ventricle into the pulmonary artery. During the insertion the inflated balloon causes the catheter tip to follow the flow of venous blood through the right heart chambers into the pulmonary artery and then into one of its branches. The inflated balloon occludes or 'wedges' the branch of the pulmonary artery. The pulmonary vascular bed beyond the balloon is directly in communication via the pulmonary vein, left atrium and the open mitral valve with the left ventricle. The pressure measured at the catheter tip in the occluded pulmonary artery therefore normally approximates to the pressure in the left ventricle during end diastole, and provides information on the function of the left ventricle as a pump. The pressure measurement is known as the *pulmonary capillary wedge pressure*. As the left ventricle deteriorates as a pump, backward passive venous congestion develops and is recorded as an increase in the pulmonary capillary wedge pressure, giving warning of decreasing cardiac output. The catheters can also be used to measure cardiac output by a thermodilution technique.

The information obtainable by the use of the Swan Ganz catheter permits hypotension due to hypovolaemia to be distinguished from pump failure (cardiogenic hypotension). The technique is not usually employed outside intensive care or cardiac units and a full description of its use is outside the scope of this book.

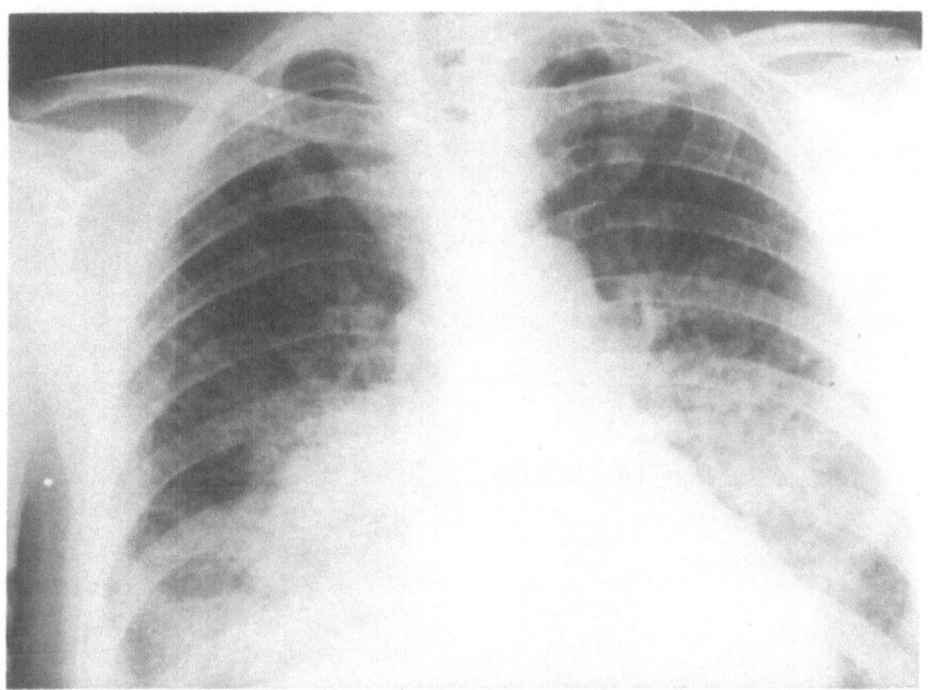

14. Radiological investigations

14.1

A *chest X-ray* is an essential investigation for most patients requiring intravenous therapy. It gives information on heart size and the lung fields. The presence or absence of the bilateral soft shadows of pulmonary oedema is of particular importance (Fig. 10). Pleural or pericardial effusions may be present.

14.2

A *plain X-ray of abdomen* may often be of help. The intestine may be distended with gas and fluid levels may be present suggesting intestinal obstruction. It may be possible to see the outlines of the kidneys, which if reduced in size suggest chronic impairment of renal function. The average size of the kidneys is 12–13 cm or $3\frac{1}{2}$ times the height of the lumbar vertebrae. Inequality in kidney size (more than 1.5 cm difference) may be present. Radio-opaque renal calculi may be seen or calcification may be present in mesenteric lymph nodes. In a recent patient admitted as an

66

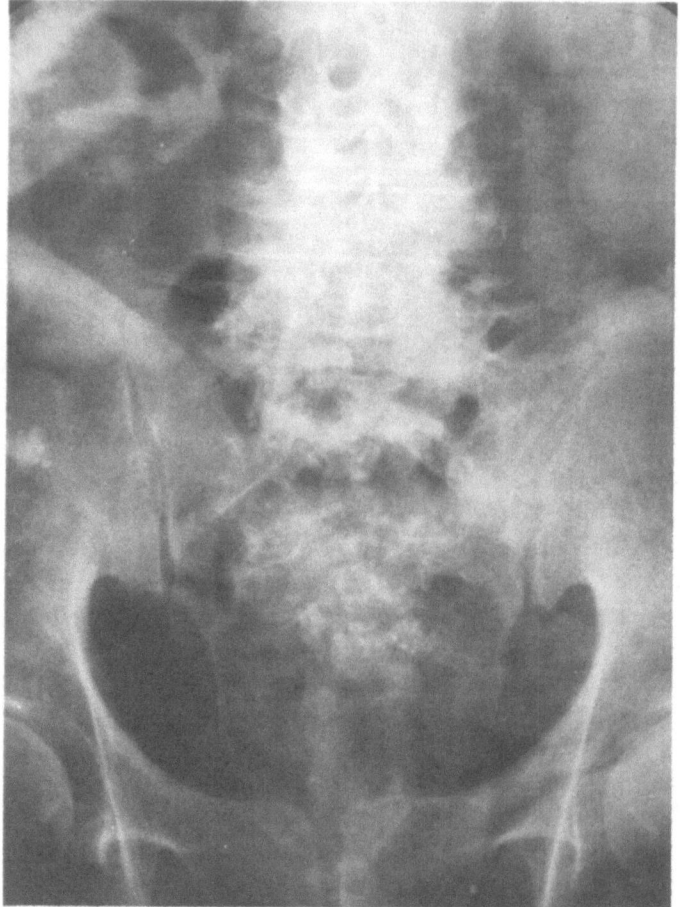

Fig. 11. Calcification in psoas abscess overlying sacral area.

emergency with a serum urea of 86 mmol/l and potassium of 8.4 mmol/l the first clue to the underlying diagnosis (obstructive uropathy due to renal tuberculosis) was given by the presence of scattered calcification in a calcified psoas abscess overlying the sacral area (Fig. 11).

References

1. Astrup P: A simple electrometric technique for the determination of carbon dioxide tension. Scand J clin lab investig 8: 33–43, 1956.
2. Rooth G: Acid–base and electrolyte balance. Chicago Year Book Medical Publishers Inc, 1974.
3. Severinghaus JW, Bradley AF: Electrodes for Po_2 and Pco_2 determination. J appl physiol 13: 515–520, 1958.
4. Sendroy J, Cecchini, LP: Determination of human body surface area from height and weight. J appl physiol 7: 1–12, 1954.
5. Dubois D, Dubois EF: Clinical calorimetry: A formula to estimate the approximate surface area if height and weight be known. Arch int med 17: 863–871, 1916.
6. Coppel DL: Monitoring and replacement of blood loss. In: Trauma Care. Odling-Smee W, Crockard A (eds.). London: Academic press. 1981, pp 163–165.

8. Solutions for intravenous therapy and their uses

Intravenous therapy is made easier by the use of simple solutions rather than mixed solutions.

There are a number of commercially available electrolyte solutions which contain most necessary ions in approximately normal proportions. These are often used by the inexperienced doctor in the belief that no harm can come from their use. However, if they are given inappropriately they use up volume and subsequent correction of electrolyte disturbances is made more difficult. Moreover, it is impossible to replete the sodium-depleted patient by giving a solution containing sodium in normal concentration.

The use of simple solutions enables a prescription to be written which is precisely tailored to the needs of the individual patient. The simple electrolyte solutions are often manufactured in the hospital pharmacy and therefore tend to be cheaper than ready prepared commercial solutions.

The prescription for intravenous fluids is intended to: (1) make up any deficiencies; (2) keep up with continuing losses.

When volume and osmolality are both reduced then osmolality should be corrected first, but of course volume will be at least partially replaced at the same time.

When an abnormality of pH is also present the solution given to correct osmolality should also restore the pH towards normal.

Before prescribing intravenous fluids it is necessary to decide the volume and the time over which it is to be given (Chapters 4 and 5).

The required volume of electrolyte-containing fluid is usually given over 12–24 hours, along with an additional 500 ml to cover insensible loss of water via respiration and the skin. In the obviously depleted patient without evidence of cardiac defeat it is usually safe to give 2/3 of the total quantity over 12 hours. The patient is then reassessed, the biochemistry repeated and note is taken of continuing loss of fluid by all routes. By this time the blood pressure if originally low should have improved, and urine should have been produced but the patient may still appear to be depleted (the original estimate was too low) and additional 1–2 litres of appropriate fluid may need to be added to the amount already planned for the second 12 hours. Following this the whole situation is again assessed and further correction prescribed for the second and likewise for the third 24-hour period, by which time very considerable clinical and biochemical improvement is to be expected.

In exceptional circumstances it may be necessary to give very large amounts of fluid rapidly. Very rapid administration of fluid should be monitored by measurement of central venous pressure. Fluid should be infused at a rate which does not elevate the central venous pressure above 10–12 cm H_2O. In shock due to sodium loss it may be necessary to give up to 2000 ml 0.9% sodium chloride per hour.

Solutions for intravenous use:

1. 5% dextrose

Water cannot be given intravenously because it causes rapid swelling and lysis of blood cells. 5% dextrose solution is approximately isotonic and is used when water is needed.

2. Sodium chloride solutions

Sodium chloride solution in a range of concentrations is used very frequently for intravenous infusion (Table 19). It may be given for treatment of the conditions shown in Table 20.

Table 19. Sodium chloride solutions for intravenous use.

Concentration W/V	Sodium mmol/l	Chloride mmol/l
0.9%	155	155
2.7%	475	475
5.0%	855	855
0.45%	77	77
0.22%	38	38

2.1. Replacement of sodium deficiency

Bearing in mind the large contribution made by sodium to osmolality of extracellular fluid, it is clear that deficiency of sodium from any cause (Chapter 11) needs to be corrected and in many circumstances sodium is given most appropriately as chloride. However, it should be remembered that sodium chloride in large amounts can cause metabolic acidosis for the following reason.

Extracellular fluid normally contains more sodium ions than chloride ions (sodium 140 mmol/l, chloride 105 mmol/l). Isotonic sodium chloride contains 155 mmol/l of sodium and of chloride. Therefore, administration of sodium chloride adds an excess of chloride ions. When kidney function is not normal the kidney cannot excrete the excess chloride. The sodium ions are excreted as sodium bicar-

Table 20. Uses of sodium chloride solution.

1. Replacement of sodium deficiency
2. Replacement of chloride deficiency
3. Correction of metabolic alkalosis
4. Acute replacement of volume in shock
5. Maintenance intravenous therapy

bonate and hydrogen is retained with the chloride ions, leading to metabolic acidosis. Large amounts of sodium chloride should not be given to patients who are already acidaemic or who have impaired renal function.

Sodium chloride in 0.9% concentration is used to replete the patient deficient in sodium and is very safe for this purpose as with reasonable care in prescribing there is little likelihood of rendering the patient hypernatraemic. The amount of sodium required is calculated from the plasma sodium level and the estimated volume of total body water of the patient (Chapter 2).

Where X is the patient's plasma sodium concentration and Y his total body water volume the calculation is as follows:

$$(140 - X) \, Y = \text{sodium deficit in mmol}$$

0.9% sodium chloride actually contains 155 mmol of sodium and 155 mmol of chloride per litre, but for the practical purpose of prescribing, the figure 150 is near enough. This approximation makes the calculation of the required volume very easy.

When an attempt has already been made to correct sodium deficiency by using an inappropriate solution, the patient may not be deficient in volume and it may be necessary to give the required amount of sodium chloride as one of the more concentrated solutions (Table 19).

The more dilute solutions of sodium chloride are used mainly in paediatric therapy. In fact I have frequently used the 0.9% sodium chloride replacement and maintenance therapy as already described for the treatment of children, the actual volumes being based on weight and age [1] (Appendix 3), and have found this satisfactory.

The most generally useful solution is 0.9% sodium chloride and it should be chosen unless there is a firm indication (such as lack of volume) to use a more concentrated or more dilute solution.

2.2. Replacement of chloride deficiency

When chloride deficiency is present there is usually a deficiency of sodium, e.g., hypochloraemic alkalosis due to vomiting/aspiration, and sodium chloride is the appropriate solution. There are rare exceptions, e.g., Conn's syndrome.

2.3. Correction of metabolic alkalosis (Chapter 17)

As already explained sodium chloride given intravenously in large amounts leads to metabolic acidosis by the chloride ions leading to hydrogen ion retention. The hydrogen ion retaining property of chloride is exploited for the correction of alkalosis. This is particularly appropriate in the commonest cause of metabolic alkalosis – the hypochloraemic alkalosis associated with severe and prolonged vomiting or aspiration of gastric contents, where chloride and sodium deficiency accompany the alkalosis.

The use of intravenous infusion of ammonium chloride is sometimes recommended for the correction of metabolic alkalosis. I have never found it necessary to resort to infusion of ammonium chloride for correction of alkalosis and find that sodium chloride is satisfactory for this purpose. This avoids the unnecessary use of the potentially toxic ammonium ion. Ammonium chloride is contra-indicated in patients with disturbed liver function in whom it may precipitate hepatic coma.

2.4. Acute replacement of volume in shock

Sodium chloride solution can be infused for hypovolaemia due to severe haemorrhage as a temporary expedient until blood or plasma can be obtained. Mixed electrolyte solutions are probably better for this purpose. In shock due to sodium and water loss it may be necessary to give up to 2 litres 0.9% saline per hour, while monitoring central venous pressure. In an average adult up to 40% of blood volume, amounting to 3–4 litres may be infused with safety. This volume eventually leads to dilution of plasma proteins and oedema, and a fall in haematocrit, which may be as low as 28%. The reduced oxygen-carrying capacity can be compensated by administering positive pressure ventilation with increased oxygen.

2.5. Maintenance intravenous therapy

Sodium chloride solution is convenient for replacing daily losses of sodium in patients who are in normal electrolyte state.

The simplest way to ensure that the patient remains in balance over days or even weeks of intravenous therapy is to base the daily prescription on the previous day's output (volumes of urine, aspirate, etc.). Over the following 24 hours this is replaced by 1/2 volume of 0.9% sodium chloride and 1/2 volume of 5% dextrose or nutritional fluid (taking into account their sodium content if any and reducing the sodium chloride appropriately). Potassium is also needed and is given as 30 mmol potassium chloride per litre output. The insensible loss of water via respiration and skin is replaced by 500 ml 5% dextrose.

The daily prescription *per litre output* is, therefore:

> 500 ml 0.9% sodium chloride + 30 mmol potassium chloride + 500 ml 5% dextrose

To this is added 500 ml 5% dextrose for insensible loss.

If it is anticipated that intravenous therapy is likely to be needed for more than a few days some of the 5% dextrose is replaced by nutritive fluid (Chapter 21).

Note that this system of maintenance therapy ignores the differences between the actual electrolyte content of urine and gastrointestinal fluids. However, in patients receiving intravenous therapy the plasma eletrolytes are determined each day and any slight deviation from normal which may occur after several days is easily corrected. This system is not suitable for the treatment of severely ill patients whose renal function may be abnormal and who require full intensive care for long periods. In such patients daily analysis of electrolyte excretion in urine and other body fluid losses should be carried out as a guide to replacement.

3. Sodium bicarbonate

Solutions containing various concentrations of sodium bicarbonate are given when it is desired to correct metabolic acidosis and there is sodium space (Chapter 3), or in more limited amount for the correction of lactic acidosis due to tissue anoxia. In the latter situation great care must be taken to avoid causing hypernatraemia and the attendant risk of cerebral haemorrhage.

Sodium bicarbonate is usually available in concentrated solution (8.4%) containing 1 mmol of sodium and of bicarbonate per 1 ml of solution. Sodium bicarbonate does not keep well in dilute solution. If a more dilute solution is required it is prepared just before use by dilution of the 8.4% concentration with 5% dextrose.

Sodium bicarbonate is given for the replacement of sodium deficiency in a patient who is acidaemic.

Since in most circumstances the sodium space (Chapter 3) is the critical factor in deciding how much sodium bicarbonate may be given with safety, the calculation is based on the patient's plasma sodium figure as described for sodium chloride.

$$(140 - X)\,Y = \text{sodium space in mmol}$$

(X being patient's plasma sodium concentration and Y the total body water)

The calculated amount of sodium is then given as the appropriate volume of sodium bicarbonate (1 mmol/1ml) diluted with 5% dextrose to the appropriate volume.

The amount of sodium bicarbonate required to correct the degree of acidaemia actually present can be calculated from the patient's plasma bicarbonate level.

$$(25 - Z)\,Y = \text{bicarbonate deficit in mmol}$$

(Z being patient's bicarbonate level and Y his total body water)

Note however, that it may be unwise to completely correct the acidaemia because of risk of causing hypernatraemia.

4. One-sixth molar sodium lactate

One-sixth molar sodium lactate which consists of equal parts of d- and l-lactate, can be used in most circumstances for the same purposes as sodium bicarbonate. It keeps well in dilute solution. The lactate ions are metabolised in the liver into bicarbonate, so that the effect is similar to giving sodium bicarbonate.

One-sixth molar sodium lactate contains 162 mmol of sodium and of lactate per litre. It is convenient of ease for prescribing to regard the 1/6 m solution as containing 150 mmol of both sodium and lactate (bicarbonate) per litre.

Sodium lactate should not be given to patients with impaired liver function or with right-sided heart failure (where hepatic function is impaired) who may be unable to metabolise lactate to bicarbonate. It is not suitable for correction of tissue acidosis after cardiac arrest where rapid correction is needed.

5. Potassium chloride

Potassium chloride is available as a solution containing 1 mmol per 1 ml. *This must always be given diluted* in other intravenous fluid. It is usually given diluted so that 1 litre of infusion contains 20–40 mmol. When severe potassium deficiency is present and there is a shortage of volume in which to dilute it, it is possible to give it in more concentrated solution. It is unwise for the inexperienced doctor to prescribe potassium in concentrations above 50 mmol/l and higher concentrations it should not be given more rapidly than 20–40 mmol/hour.

Potassium chloride can be given in concentrations as high as 80 mmol/l, with ECG monitoring, by a doctor experienced in its use.

It is often stated that potassium should not be given intravenously until there is an 'adequate' urinary output. Patients with potassium deficiency associated with hypochloraemic alkalosis due to vomiting/aspiration often have oliguria. Both sodium chloride and potassium chloride are needed for correction of this abnormality and rapid improvement in urinary volume follows intravenous infusion of potassium chloride diluted in 0.9% saline.

As the plasma concentration of potassium does not give a true indication of intracellular potassium status, and intracellular potassium is not measured in clinical laboratories, the amount needed is decided on general principles (Chapter 15). It is often helpful to determine the 24-hour excretion of potassium. It should be remembered that a normal serum potassium level in a patient with acidosis (which causes potassium to move out of cells) indicates considerable potassium loss. Therefore the acid-base situation must be taken into consideration. The patient with hypochloraemic alkalosis due to vomiting may be deficient by 250 mmol or more despite a normal serum potassium concentration. In acidotic patients with a low serum potassium concentration much more than this may be needed.

6. Potassium acetate

This is used for patients in whom potassium deficiency is associated with acidosis, for example in treatment of severe hyperchloraemic acidosis with potassium deficiency associated with urinary diversion operations. The acetate is metabolised to bicarbonate in the liver, and helps with the correction of the acidosis.

It is available in ampoules containing 3 mmol of potassium and of acetate per 1 ml. *This must be given diluted* in other intravenous solutions, in the same way as potassium chloride.

7. Magnesium sulphate

This is used for the treatment of hypomagnesaemia and sometimes to reduce cerebral oedema in eclampsia (Chapter 20). Magnesium sulphate is available in 10% solution (10 g in 100 ml) and 50% solution (50 g in 100 ml). The 10% solution contains 4 mmol of magnesium and of sulphate in 10 ml, the 50% solution 20 mmol of magnesium and of sulphate in 10 ml.

8. Isotonic mixed electrolyte solutions

These include Ringer's lactate solution, Hartmann's solution, Darrow's solution and many others. A list of contents of some of the commoner solutions is given in Table 21.

The reasons for preferring simple solutions for most purposes have already been stated. However, mixed isotonic solutions are useful as vehicles for intravenous administration of drugs during anaesthesia. They can also be used to replace volume in situations of shock associated with rapid volume loss (haemorrhage) until colloid solutions can be obtained, and are probably preferable to 0.9% sodium chloride for this purpose. Appendix 4 contains general guidance on intravenous administration of drugs.

9. Colloidal solutions

These are used for expanding circulating blood volume when shock is present. Most of these solutions (Table 22) are retained within the vascular compartment and

Table 21. Isotonic mixed electrolyte solutions.

Solutions	Na^+	K^+	Cl^-	HCO_3^-	Ca^{++}	Mg^{++}	CHO
Hartmann's	131	2	111	29 (acetate)	2	–	none or 5% dextrose
Ringer's lactate	129	5	111	27 (lactate)	1.5	–	none or 5% dextrose
Darrow's	121	35	103	53 (lactate)	–	–	none or 5% dextrose
Plasmalyte 148	140	5	98	50 (acetate 27 gluconate 23)	–	1.5	5% dextrose
Plasmalyte 148 in water	140	5	98	50 (acetate 27 gluconate 23)	–	1.5	–
Plasmalyte 50/30	150	30	67	24 (acetate 12 lactate 12)	3.0	2.5	–

Table 22. Colloidal solutions.

---

1. Whole blood
2. Packed red blood cells
3. Pooled plasma
4. Plasma protein fraction
5. Concentrated salt-poor albumen
6. Dextran

---

increase the vascular osmotic pressure, leading to further improvement in blood volume by drawing in water from extracellular fluid.

9.1. Whole blood

This is the most suitable fluid for the treatment of shock due to haemorrhage. There is inevitably some delay in obtaining cross-matched blood but this is minimised in intensive care units accustomed to treating patients with severe trauma.

It can be estimated that 1 unit of blood will raise the haemoglobin level about 1 g/dl.

Whole blood may contain hepatitis B antigen and as the incubation period for this is 6 weeks to 6 months, jaundice occurring within 6 months after transfusion should be regarded as suspect and treated in isolation while appropriate tests for the antigen are carried out. This risk is of great importance in dialysis units where the same patients return over long periods for repeated treatments, and where transfusion may be required on many occasions and where spillage of patients' blood may occur from time to time. The risk has been reduced by the introduction of routine testing for hepatitis B antigen of all blood used for transfusion. In the United Kingdom a special code of practice has been drawn up in an attempt to minimise the special risks of hepatitis B in dialysis units.

Incompatible transfusion is followed by fever, loin pain, oliguria or anuria and acute renal failure. It may occasionally occur even when the blood has been cross-matched and appears to be compatible.

A commoner cause of incompatible transfusion is failure to check carefully that the blood is given to the patient for whom it has been cross-matched.

I recall a patient who required transfusion after a post-partum haemorrhage who was given 2 units of cross-matched apparently compatible blood. She appeared well the evening of transfusion but the following morning had a mild fever, and was thought to be slightly jaundiced. She passed a small amount of dark coloured urine that morning and thereafter remained anuric for 17 days. Further investigation showed that the blood given had been incompatible for the Kell antigen. She required haemodialysis four times and in all was given 12 units of blood. A 2-hour cross-match was used and the blood was screened for the Kell antigen and a total of 250 units had to be tested to find the 12 units used.

Transient fever after blood transfusion may be due to bacterial contamination or allergic reaction.

Young females requiring transfusion should be given Rh matched or Rh negative blood to avoid possible sensitisation to the rhesus antigen.

Over-transfusion with whole blood may cause acute pulmonary oedema. This may develop during the transfusion or within an hour or two afterwards. This should be treated by immediate venesection and removal of 200–400 ml of blood unless the signs of overload are minimal, when 40 mg frusemide intravenously may suffice.

Stored blood contains potassium in increased concentration because of lysis of red cells, and when massive transfusion is required elevation of the patient's plasma potassium may occur. The citrate used as anticoagulant may lead to hypocalcaemia after large transfusions. Both potassium and calcium concentration should be monitored when large amounts of blood are infused.

9.2. Packed red blood cells

Packed cells are prepared by centrifuging whole blood and withdrawing most of the plasma. Packed red cells are particularly useful for transfusion of patients with poor tolerance of a fluid load or sodium, such as patients with renal failure or who have recently been in left ventricular failure.

There is an increasing tendency to conserve the use of blood by using packed red cells for patients for whom whole blood is not specially requested. The plasma obtained is then available for use when red cells are not needed. Platelets may also be separated and used for platelet transfusion.

The hazards of transfusion of packed cells are similar to those associated with the use of whole blood.

9.3. Pooled plasma

This is a good expander of the circulating blood volume because there is no need for typing and cross-match. However, there is a risk of contamination with hepatitis B antigen.

9.4. Plasma protein fraction

Plasma protein fraction has been treated with heat to destroy hepatitis B antigen and is now generally preferred to pooled plasma.

9.5. Concentrated salt-poor albumen

This is prepared by concentration and desalination of plasma albumen. It is used for patients with very low plasma albumen concentrations due to urinary protein loss or to cirrhosis.

9.6. Dextran

Dextran is an artificial plasma substitute which is produced by polymerization of glucose. Polymers of molecular weight of 40,000, 70,000, 110,000 and 150,000 are available. They are given as a colloidal suspension which remains in the blood stream for some hours and increases the oncotic pressure as does albumen infusion. Up to 2 litres may be infused over one hour. Part of the infused dextran is excreted by the kidneys within 24 hours and the remainder is metabolized.

Dextran 40 has a shorter effect than the higher molecular weight dextrans as it is excreted fairly rapidly by the kidneys (50% within 3 hours). It is used to improve peripheral blood flow in ischaemic disease of limbs.

Dextran 70 and the higher molecular weight dextrans are used mainly for volume expansion, especially in the treatment of burns. They should not be used to replace haemorrhage, when blood is more appropriate, or water and electrolyte losses.

Dextran in any form must be used with discretion because it dilutes the haemoglobin and may lead to a serious degree of anaemia and thus anoxia. Great caution is necessary when giving it to a patient who is already anaemic.

All forms of dextran may lead to prolonged bleeding time because of dilution of fibrinogen and clotting factors.

Hypersensitivity reactions are fairly common with both forms of dextran and include urticaria, nausea, bronchial spasm, hypotension and shock. If symptoms and signs suggesting allergic reaction develop the infusion should be discontinued at once and an antihistamine given.

Acute renal failure, with renal tubular swelling on biopsy, has been reported following infusion of low molecular weight dextran. Four cases of acute renal failure occurred in our orthopaedic wards within the first few months after a policy of post-operative infusion of low molecular weight dextran was adapted for prophylaxis against deep venous thrombosis. A reason for the acute renal failure other than the dextran infusion was not found. In all the patients the renal failure was of short duration and recovered with conservative treatment without dialysis.

Low molecular dextran or perhaps indeed any from of dextran, should be avoided in patients known to have impaired renal function. Underhydration must be avoided and the renal function must be carefully monitored over the next few days.

10. Nutritive solutions

Intravenous nutrition and the various solutions available will be discussed in Chapter 21.

11. Ammonium chloride

This has been advocated for the treatment of metabolic alkalosis. The reasons for preferring sodium chloride for this purpose have been discussed.

It is available as 0.9% (isotonic) solution for intravenous use.

12. Mannitol

Mannitol is available as 5, 10, 15 and 20% solutions. It is given as an osmotic diuretic (Chapter 1). When given intravenously it produces a rapid increase in plasma osmolality. Water is drawn from extracellular fluid and cells into the vascular compartment, leading to a fall in plasma sodium.

Mannitol is sometimes given intravenously during surgery which may lead to shock, in the hope that it may prevent acute renal failure by increasing renal blood flow and causing an osmotic diuresis, the usual dose being 50 to 100 g. It is also used in the hope of aborting incipient renal failure in patients who are already oliguric. Convincing evidence that it is effective for either of these purposes is lacking, and in the great majority of such patients improvement in urinary output follows improvement in blood pressure and restoration of any deficiency of water and electrolyte which may be present. In patients in whom the cardiovascular system is already compromised, or who has already been volume expanded, infusion of mannitol may precipitate acute pulmonary oedema, and very careful observation is needed.

Mannitol has been used as an osmotic diuretic following poisoning, as 5% or 10% solution.

Mannitol is sometimes used to lower intracranial pressure in cerebral oedema.

13. Forced diuresis

Forced diuresis may be used to increase excretion of certain drugs after overdose, e.g., salicylates, barbiturates, amphetamine. Following overdosage of some drugs such as salicylate where there is a marked tendency to acidosis a forced alkaline diuresis is used.

It is important to remember that overdosage of salicylate and other drugs may cause acute renal failure. It is essential to measure urinary output per hour and ensure that the intravenous infusion does not get more than 1.5 litres ahead of the urinary output. A central venous manometer is helpful but not essential.

The following regimen if used with due care is quite safe and can be used with $\frac{1}{2}$ volumes for the treatment of young children.

1. Pass urethral catheter
2. Infuse 1.5 litres 5% dextrose over $1\frac{1}{2}$ hours
3. Give 40 mg frusemide intravenously as soon as infusion is commenced
4. Provided urine is passed in reasonable quantity during this first infusion, proceed with forced diuresis
5. Over each 2 hour period give
   500 ml 0.9% sodium chloride + 15 mmol KCl
   500 ml 5% dextrose + 15 mmol KCl
6. Repeat 40 mg frusemide intravenously every 4–6 hours according to response
7. Collect urine in 12-hour aliquots for estimation of toxin thought to be present
8. Estimate urea and electrolytes every 12 hours
9. If able to swallow, allow 500 ml of fluids orally, otherwise give 500 ml 5% dextrose intravenously *once* over each 24-hour period to cover insensible loss by respiration and skin
10. If it is necessary to use forced alkaline diuresis over each 2-hour period give:
    350 ml M/6 lactate   + 15 mmol KCl
    150 ml 0.9% sodium chloride
    500 ml 5% dextrose + 15 mmol KCl
    Proceed otherwise as above

Reference

1. Carré IJ: The management of intravenous fluid and electrolyte therapy in children. Ir J med Sc, 135–146, 1965.

9. Water loss syndrome

Synonyms: dehydration, dessication, underhydration

Reduction of body water in theory may arise from reduction in intake or increase in loss. In practice reduction in intake is complicated by continuing water loss, leading to increasing dryness or *dessication*. *Dehydration* is an appropriate term for the description of water deficiency, but this term is often used to describe the much commoner situation of loss of both water and sodium. The term water loss syndrome avoids this source of confusion.

Disturbances involving water balance alone are comparatively rare. In the majority of clinical situations abnormalities of water and sodium balance occur together. Nevertheless separate consideration of disturbances involving water and sodium is helpful for the understanding of the more common mixed disorders.

1. Pure deprivation of water

Pure deprivation of water as occurs in desert castaways is followed by increasing dessication as loss of water continues through the lungs and skin and the obligatory loss in the urine to carry the solutes which must be excreted. Some sodium is lost in sweat but this is quantitatively insignificant compared with the water loss. The water loss leads to increasing concentration of the extracellular sodium and hence to elevation of extracellular osmolality. The increased osmolality stimulates secretion of antidiuretic hormone leading to maximum concentration of urine, but the daily minimum obligatory urine volume amounts to about 400 mls. As the osmolality of extracellular fluid increases, water is withdrawn from cells so that in turn intracellular osmolality rises. Eventually the hyperosmolality of brain cells leads to disruption of brain function with hallucinations followed by coma and death.

Deprivation of water may occur in the elderly and feeble when living alone, or even in hospital if the patient is unable to reach and drink unaided, fluids placed on the bedside locker.

2. Increased water loss

Increased water loss becomes harmful only when insufficient is given to replace the loss. Causes of increased water loss are shown in Table 23. With the exception of

Table 23. Causes of increased water loss.

1. Polyuria due to impaired renal function
2. Pyelonephritis
3. Hypokalaemia
4. Hyperosmolar states
5. Excess solute administration
6. Hypercalcaemia
7. Diabetes insipidus with water deprivation
8. Lithium treatment with water deprivation
9. Repeated angiography
10. Artificial ventilation without humidification

artificial ventilation these situations are due to increase in renal clearance of free water (Chapter 1).

2.1. Polyuria due to renal impairment

In severe reduction of renal function the marked increase in nitrogenous substances in plasma leads to hyperosmolality with withdrawal of water from cells, some of which is then lost with the increased solute load diuresis. Such patients are dependent on a high urine volume to excrete excess solute, and when deprived of fluid, for example to carry out intravenous pyelography, or for a urinary concentration test, the uraemia rapidly worsens and acute renal failure may be superimposed on the chronic condition. When an intravenous pyelogram is needed in a patient with considerable impairment of renal function, the patient should be normally hydrated, and a higher dose of contrast medium given. If the patient is oedematous, ultrasound examination may be preferable as high dose pyelography entails giving a considerable sodium load.

2.2. Pyelonephritis

Patients with chronic pyelonephritis often have impaired tubular function and are unable to concentrate their urine, leading to loss of free water.

2.3. Hypokalaemia

Chronic hypokalaemia causes loss of renal ability to concentrate the urine with consequent polyuria (Chapter 15).

2.4. Hyperosmolar coma

At normal levels blood glucose contributes very little to plasma osmolality. Very high levels of plasma glucose may occasionally develop in patients with diabetes mellitus, more often in elderly patients. As the plasma glucose reaches high levels the osmolality of extracellular fluid greatly exceeds that of intracellular water, with the result that water is lost from cells into extracellular fluid. The high concentration of glucose being filtered at the glomeruli results in osmotic diuresis (Chapter 1) and a large loss of water. This in turn leads to elevation in the plasma concentration of sodium and further increase in extracellular osmolality and further cellular dehydration.

2.5. Excess solute administration

Administration of excessive solutes with insufficient water can lead to an osmotic diuresis and loss of free water. Nasogastric feeding of an unconscious patient, especially with high protein foods in a small volume of water, produces a solute load of nitrogenous products. Similar circumstances arise in a patient with a bleeding peptic ulcer, where the blood provides a protein meal and milk and little water may be given as treatment.

2.6. Hypercalcaemia

Hypercalcaemia (due to hyperparathyroidism, metastatic malignancy, myelomatosis, vitamin D intoxication, or ectopic production of parathyroid hormone by tumour) can lead to increased plasma osmolality, osmotic diuresis and cellular dehydration. This situation arises only with very high levels of serum calcium – 3.2 mmol/l and above.

2.7. Diabetes insipidus with water deprivation

This is due to failure of production or release of antidiuretic hormone in response to a rise in plasma osmolality. Primary diabetes insipidus is rare but the secondary type is fairly common. It may follow trauma to the head or surgery to the hypothalamic/pituitary region of the brain or be due to a tumour, cyst or granuloma (for example, sarcoidosis) in this area. There is, therefore, an obligatory high urine volume leading to increasing thirst, both continuing by night as well as by day. The osmolality of the urine is usually below 200 mosmol/l. In normal circumstances, the thirst mechanism ensures that plasma osmolality is kept within the normal range or just above it. If the patient is deprived of his usual high water intake, for example if unconscious, the plasma sodium and therefore the osmolality rapidly rises.

2.8. Lithium treatment with water deprivation

Patients who are given lithium for recurrent manic depressive illness may develop a diabetes insipidus-like syndrome if they are deprived of fluids, for example in preparation for operation. High urinary volume leads to dehydration, followed by decreased excretion of lithium and symptoms of lithium toxicity (malaise, tremor, dysarthria) in addition to those of dehydration. As lithium is now widely prescribed this may become a common cause of dehydration.

2.9. Repeated angiography

The high dose of contrast material used in angiography, especially if given as a sodium salt, can if repeated within a short time interval provide a significant increase in plasma osmolality and cause osmotic loss of fluid.

2.10. Artificial ventilation without humidification

Large amounts of water may be lost during artificial ventilation, especially if a tracheostomy is present, if the respiratory gases are not humidified. Humidification is now used routinely. It should be remembered that use of humidification reduces the insensible loss of water to about 200 ml rather than the usual 500 ml.

3. Physical signs of water loss

With minor degrees of water loss, although the patient may complain of thirst on physical examination he may appear normal.

As water deficiency becomes more marked the skin feels dry, including the axilla and groin. The temperature may rise. The tongue becomes dry, red and fissured, and may become so swollen that speech becomes difficult. The dryness of the mucous membranes is obvious to the touch.

In pure water loss the skin turgor is normal or nearly so.

4. Laboratory findings of water loss

With minor degrees of water loss the movement of water from cells into intracellular fluid at first prevents any change in blood chemistry. As water continues to be lost, haemoconcentration occurs, the serum sodium concentration and haemotocrit (packed cell volume) rise. The haemocrit may be above 50% (normal 47% $\pm$ 5% in males, 42% $\pm$ 5% in females) and the serum sodium is usually above 150 mmol/l.

5. Treatment of water loss syndrome

The treatment of water loss is to give water. In the conscious patient in whom there is no contra-indication to use of the gastrointestinal tract this is best done by the oral route. If the patient is unable or unwilling to drink water it may be given by a nasogastric tube. Fluid must *not* be given by nasogastric tube in an unconscious patient unless a cuffed endotrachael tube has been inserted to prevent fluid getting into the lungs. If it is necessary to use the intravenous route, pure water cannot be given as the red cells absorb water and undergo haemolysis. It must be given as an isotonic solution such as 5% dextrose.

6. Amount of water required

The amount of water given should replace the water deficit and allow for continuing loss by urine, respiration and sweat.

Knowledge of the body weight is helpful in making an estimate of the volume of water needed.

In the conscious patient who complains of thirst, but clinical signs of underhydration are minimal, the water deficit is about 2% of the body weight. A 70-kg man would, therefore, need about 1400 ml to which should be added 1500 ml for the daily production of urine and losses in respiration and sweat.

If there are marked clinical signs of underhydration, the urinary output may be low (though not if the cause is excessive urinary loss). Marked thirst may be present. The water deficit is about 6% of body weight. The deficit of water is, therefore, about 4200 ml for a 70-kg man.

If in addition to marked signs of underhydration the patient is confused or delirious the water deficit is in excess of 7% of body weight, or over 5 litres in a 70-kg man.

In more severe cases of water loss it is usually safer to replace the water deficit over two days, on each day giving half the estimated deficit plus approximately 1500 ml for current losses. Rapid correction may cause cerebral oedema.

The serum electrolytes should be measured twice daily. It may become obvious that sodium and perhaps potassium have been lost as well as water and in any case replacement of current loss of these ions will be needed. This is given as half of the volume of measured urine as 0.9% saline, accompanied by 30 mmol potassium chloride per litre. The other half is given as 5% dextrose as is the replacement for insensible fluid loss (about 500 ml).

10. Water excess syndrome

Synonym: overhydration

When the kidneys, heart, hypothalamus and adrenals are normal it is almost impossible to take enough water by mouth to produce overhydration. However, it can be achieved by a psychotic patient – compulsive water drinking or psychogenic polydipsia. Increased water intake in the normal subject leads to dilution of extracellular water and therefore a fall in osmolality. This inhibits the release of ADH and is followed by excretion of an increased volume of dilute urine.

1. Water excess caused by intravenous infusion

Overhydration can be produced by intravenous infusion of water (as 5% dextrose) at very fast rates even when the kidneys, heart and hypothalamus is normal. Intravenous infusion of 5% dextrose even at normal rates can produce overhydration in a variety of clinical circumstances (Table 24) and must be used with discretion.

Table 24. Situations in which intravenous infusion of 5% dextrose may lead to water excess.

1. Acute renal failure
2. Severe congestive heart failure
3. Cirrhosis of liver
4. Syndrome of inappropriate secretion of anti-diuretic hormone (SIADH)

1.1. Acute renal failure

Overhydration is a common finding in patients with acute renal failure. It may be several days before the medical staff notice that the urinary output has fallen to a very low level and during this time fluids will have been given as if urine production was normal. This situation can be avoided if careful fluid balance charts are kept (and noted by the medical staff) in all patients who are acutely ill, hypotensive, and post-operatively if hypotension occurs. Hypotension leads to reduced renal blood flow and oliguria, but even if urinary output improves in 24–48 hours, as often happens, too much fluid may have been given, specially in the elderly patient with poor cardiac reserve.

1.2. Severe congestive heart failure

Renal blood flow is reduced in congestive heart failure, leading to reduction in urinary output and reduced need for water.

1.3. Cirrhosis of the liver

Renal blood flow is often reduced in patients with cirrhosis. Decreased peripheral resistance is probably the main factor leading to hypotension or at least relatively low blood pressure. The renal blood flow appears to be shunted to the medullary region reducing glomerular filtration. Many patients have hypoalbuminaemia. Patients with cirrhosis may, therefore, be very susceptible to water excess.

1.4. Syndrome of inappropriate secretion of anti-diuretic hormone (SIADH)

Conditions of stress lead to increased secretion of ADH. These include fear, pain, trauma, major or even minor surgery, acute severe infection. In most of these situations excess secretion of ADH is of fairly short duration, up to 36 hours but occasionally it may last longer. Many drugs lead to excess production of ADH, of particular importance are anaesthetic and analgesic drugs because they are used in circumstances in which hypotension and reduced renal blood flow are also common. Cerebral lesions in the region of the hypothalamus and pituitary may lead to SIADH. Tumours of many types have been described as leading to SIADH, the first to be described and probably the commonest, being oat cell carcinoma of the lung. Some of the numerous conditions reported in association with SIADH are listed in Table 25.

It should be noted that SIADH is *not* due to excess water intake, but its presence makes the patient very susceptible to water excess.

The patient with SIADH does *not* have oedema or hypotension. The plasma sodium and osmolality are reduced. Urinary excretion of sodium continues despite the low plasma sodium concentration, and the urinary osmolality usually exceeds the plasma osmolality. The renal function is normal and adrenal malfunction can be excluded by the presence of normal levels of plasma aldosterone and urinary excretion of aldosterone.

2. Water excess caused by irrigation

During resection of the prostate by the transurethral route large volumes of 1.5% glycine in water may be used to irrigate the prostate bed. Both glycine and water are absorbed. Severe dilutional hyponatraemia may result either immediately after

Table 25. Conditions associated with SIADH.

---

1. *Stress*
   fear
   pain
   operation
   anaesthesia
   acute infection
2. *Cerebral lesions*
   trauma
   space-occupying lesions
   vascular accident
   infections
3. *Tumors*
   lung
   gastrointestinal tract
   prostrate
   lymphoma
   thymoma
4. *Chronic pulmonary infection*
   tuberculosis
   aspergillosis
   abscess
5. *Drugs*
   cyclophosphamide
   chlorpropamide
   indomethacin
   clofibrate
   barbiturates
   vincristine
6. *Positive pressure ventilation*

---

surgery or 24–48 hours later. The absorption of large amounts of glycine leads to increased excretion of oxalate and glycolate which may also be hazardous.

3. Symptoms and signs of water excess

The symptoms vary according to how rapidly the water load has occurred. If the onset is very rapid, confusion, delirium, inco-ordination, convulsions and breathlessness dominate the picture. When the accumulation of water has occurred more slowly the patient may complain of weakness, headache, muscle twitching, nausea and may vomit before developing confusion and bizarre behaviour. If the patient has been weighed, weight gain will have occurred.

The skin feels warm and moist. There may be oedema on the skin which can be demonstrated by rolling the fihger over an area of subcutaneous bone when a fingerprint will be formed.

Water excess should be considered when a post-operative patient behaves strangely, has a convulsion or becomes comatose.

4. Laboratory findings

The serum sodium is characteristically low but this of itself does not prove that water excess is present, as a low serum sodium can result from true sodium loss (Chapter 11) or in certain situations in diabetic and uraemic patients. A low serum osmolality occurs *only* when water in excess of sodium is present.

The haematocrit and the mean corpuscular haemoglobin concentration are reduced when water excess is present.

5. Treatment of water excess

If the patient is not already convulsing or in coma, withholding fluid for 24 hours or longer may be all that is necessary.

When the patient is already in coma it may be life-saving to give hypertonic sodium solution intravenously. Hypertonic sodium chloride (5%) is usually given but if the patient is acidotic, then half molar sodium lactate is used. Unless the patient has become water overloaded because of failure to recognise acute renal failure, a small volume of hypertonic sodium solution will lead to excretion of large amounts of urine.

The amount of hypertonic solution is calculated as 6 ml per kg body weight, which should raise the serum sodium by approximately 10 mmol/l. It should be given at a rate of not more than 100 ml per hour.

If there is room for doubt as to whether the low serum sodium is due to water excess, one third to one half of the calculated amount should be given, the patient observed for clinical improvement and the serum electrolytes rechecked.

11. Sodium loss syndrome

Synonyms: sodium deficiency, sodium depletion, pure salt depletion, desalting water loss

Hyponatraemia means a low serum sodium concentration but has causes other than sodium loss. The term dehydration should be reserved for pure water loss. Sodium loss syndrome is the most explicit term.

Loss of sodium from the extracellular compartment leads to a fall in osmolality of extracellular fluid. Water is therefore drawn into cells with corresponding reduction in extracellular volume. If the fall in extracellular volume is sufficiently large or occurs rapidly the fall in circulating blood volume (as part of extracellular volume) leads to fall in blood pressure and shock. Shock due to sodium loss does not respond to pressor agents but rapidly responds to infusion of hypertonic sodium solution.

Sodium loss is usually, but not invariably, associated with water loss. Loss of both sodium and water is encountered much more frequently than pure water loss. When the loss is rapid, severe shock and hypotension may occur. Potassium loss often accompanies sodium loss, and potassium must be given as well as sodium in these circumstances. For the electrolyte content of gastrointestinal fluids see Chapper 4.

1. Causes of sodium loss syndrome

The causes of sodium loss are listed in Table 26.

Table 26. Causes of sodium loss syndrome.

---

1. Vomiting/aspiration
2. Diarrhoeal causes
3. Gastrointestinal and biliary fistulae
4. Loss through intact skin
5. Loss through damaged skin
6. Sequestration of extracellular fluid
7. Intrinsic renal disease
8. Adrenocortical insufficiency
9. Diabetic keto-acidosis
10. Paracentesis or acupuncture
11. Drug-induced sodium loss
12. Bartter's syndrome

1.1. Vomiting/aspiration

This is a very common cause of sodium loss. Patients vomit at home, may vomit or have gastric aspiration in hospital.

The amount of gastric fluid lost by vomiting is usually not known because of vomitus being lost over bedding or on the floor. Aspirated gastrointestinal fluid is usually measured.

Water, hydrogen ion, chloride and potassium are lost along with sodium. Hydrogen ion moves out of cells to buffer extracellular bicarbonate and potassium moves into cells to replete intracellular hydrogen loss. The volume depletion due to sodium and water loss stimulates aldosterone secretion leading to increased renal excretion of potassium. The chloride depletion also stimulates renal excretion of potassium.

The characteristic electrolyte disturbance of vomiting/aspiration is therefore hypokalaemic hypochloraemic alkalosis. When very gross depletion has occurred oliguria ensues and the serum urea rises. At this stage the serum potassium is misleadingly normal.

Example of electrolyte disturbance associated with severe vomiting.

	mmol/l
Sodium	120
Potassium	3.8
Chloride	75
Bicarbonate	40
Urea	25

1.1.1. Treatment of electrolyte disturbance due to vomiting/aspiration.

An estimate of the deficiency in volume is made from the clinical history, any measurements which may have been made, from the appearance of the skin fold and mucous membranes, and from the eyeball tension. If the skin fold (Chapter 5) remains up for 5 seconds in an adult there is a deficiency of at least 3 litres. To this should be added volume to allow for continuing aspiration (if this is present) and for insensible loss via skin and respiration, and urine, say about 2 litres. The electrolyte deficiency should therefore be given in 5 litres of solution over the ensuing 24 hours.

The sodium deficit is estimated by subtracting the observed plasma sodium concentration from the normal value and multiplying by the estimate of total body water (Chapter 8) on the basis of weight or estimated weight, say 40 litres.

Example:

$$\text{Sodium deficit} = (140–120)40 \, \text{mmol}$$
$$= 20 \times 40 \, \text{mmol}$$
$$= 800 \, \text{mmol}$$

As the plasma chloride is low (75 mmol in the example) sodium should be given as sodium chloride, and bicarbonate, which is already high, is *not* required. Five litres of 0.9% sodium chloride (1 litre contains approximately 150 mmol of sodium and chloride) contains 750 mmol sodium and chloride, which is close enough to the estimated requirement. However, potassium has also been lost but there is no direct measurement of the amount needed as the plasma level is *not* a reflection of the total body potassium as explained already. From experience, however, it is necessary to give at least 200–250 mmol/l potassium chloride when the deficiency of sodium and chloride are of this degree. The addition of 40 mmol of potassium chloride (1 ml contains 1 mmol) to each 1 litre of sodium chloride (making sure that mixing has been thorough), will give 200 mmol potassium in the 24 hours.

It is safer to err on the side of under-correction rather than risk over-correction. In fact the estimate almost always errs on the side of being too low and there is little danger of over-correction.

After the first 24 hours there should be marked clinical improvement, with increase in blood pressure and urinary output. The electrolyte concentrations in plasma, while improved, almost always still show considerable deficiency of sodium and chloride, the bicarbonate still elevated and the plasma potassium level will have fallen from its previously normal or near normal level, despite the considerable amount of potassium given, because of potassium re-entering cells. A second correction is calculated in the same way and given over 24 hours as before. It is necessary to make allowance for the urine volume (which should have increased) and the volume of aspirate, if any, plus 500 ml for insensible loss. For practical purposes, since there will be daily estimates of urea and electrolytes for guidance, it is sufficient to give half of the combined volumes of urine and vomitus as 0.9% saline, the other half being given as 5% dextrose, plus 30 mmol potassium chloride per litre of urine and vomitus. The allowance for insensible loss is given as 5% dextrose.

If the deficiency of water has been corrected already without supplying sufficient sodium it may be necessary to give more concentrated solutions of sodium chloride (Chapter 8). An estimate of volume required is made and the appropriate strength of sodium chloride is chosen.

When necessary, potassium chloride can be given in greater concentrations than 30 mmol/l, 40, 50 mmol/l or even higher concentrations being given more slowly, over the 24-hour period.

1.2. Diarrhoeal causes

Diarrhoea due to gastroenteritis, dysentery, cholera, ulcerative colitis, pseudomembranous colitis, excessive purgation, all lead to loss of sodium and water. Enormous losses occur in the watery stools of cholera. Potassium, bicarbonate and chloride are also lost. The loss of bicarbonate predominates over the loss of chloride and the electrolyte picture is one of acidosis, with a reduced plasma potassium, i.e., hyperchloraemic hypokalaemic acidosis.

1.2.1. Treatment of diarrhoeal loss

An estimate of the deficit of volume is made from the history, any measurements available, and the appearances of skin, mucous membranes and eyeball tension, as before. The sodium deficit is calculated as for vomiting but is given as sodium bicarbonate (8.4%: 1 mmol/1 ml) appropriately diluted with 5% dextrose to the volume needed, or as sodium lactate (M/6 lactate: 150 mmol/l). Potassium is given mixed with the sodium bicarbonate or lactate at a concentration of 30–40 mmol/l. The fluid is given over 24 hours as before, and a second correction given as necessary during the second 24 hours.

1.3. Gastrointestinal and biliary fistulae

Very large amounts of sodium may be lost from fistulae, especially from a pancreatic or biliary fistula. Large amounts of water, bicarbonate and potassium are also lost.

The characteristic biochemical findings are reduction in the plasma sodium, bicarbonate and potassium concentration.

1.3.1. Treatment of sodium loss via fistula

An estimate of the volume and sodium deficit is made as before. The calculated sodium deficit is given as sodium bicarbonate (8.4%: 1 mmol/1 ml) suitably diluted with 5% dextrose to volume estimated, or as sodium lactate (M/6: 150 mmol/l). Potassium is given mixed with the sodium bicarbonate or lactate in a concentration of 30–40 mmol/l. The amount calculated is given over 24 hours, along with a suitable allowance for insensible loss, and a second correction as necessary on the basis of the electrolyte concentrations, during the second 24 hours.

1.4. Loss through intact skin

The insensible loss of water through intact skin contains very little sodium but visible sweat contains 30–70 mmol/l of sodium and chloride. The loss of water by sweat causes thirst and if water is drunk in copious amounts, without salt, the plasma sodium concentration falls further by dilution by the water taken. If severe, the patient may complain of muscle cramps and the blood pressure may fall leading to shock. This situation is commonly described as *heat exhaustion*.

The sweat of patients suffering from cystic fibrosis contains abnormally large amounts of sodium – in fact the elevated sodium content of sweat is valuable in the diagnosis of this condition. Patients with cystic fibrosis are very susceptible to heat exhaustion in hot climates.

1.4.1. Treatment of heat exhaustion

Salt and water should be given by mouth until the patient feels better. In the shocked patient rapid intravenous infusion of 1 litre 0.9% sodium chloride over 1–2 hours should produce improvement. Further infusion on the basis of the electrolyte results can be given as required.

1.5. Loss through damaged skin

Very large amounts of sodium and water may be lost through skin with exudative conditions such as generalised pustular psoriasis, exudative dermatitis and 'wet' burns.

1.5.1. Treatment of loss through skin

The loss can be measured by the loss of weight in daily weighing. This gives the volume, and the sodium deficit is calculated as before from the fall in plasma sodium concentration. The sodium requirement is given as sodium chloride.

1.6. Sequestration of extracellular fluid

Extracellular fluid may accumulate in areas of damaged tissue, for example in blistering within burned areas, areas of extensive dissection in surgery, or in dilated small bowel. This is sometimes called 'third space' loss.

The loss occurs insidiously and may be undetected until large amounts have been sequestered and the blood pressure falls with the development of tachycardia. It is important to keep the possibility in mind in patients who may be at risk, for example during the development of paralytic ileus.

1.6.1. Treatment of sequestration of extracellular fluid

The fluid lost is virtually extracellular fluid and the concentrations of the plasma electrolytes remain normal but the haemoglobin concentration may rise. An appropriate solution for repletion is Hartmann's solution (Chapter 8). The quantity needed has to be estimated on the basis of the physical examination, loss of skin turgor, etc. As there is no external loss of fluid the patient's weight does not change.

1.7. Intrinsic renal disease

In the majority of patients with impaired renal function loss of sodium through the kidneys remains normal but occasional patients with chronic pyelonephritis or with polycystic disease lose very large amounts of sodium. During the recovery (diuretic) phase following acute renal failure, and after relief of urinary obstruction there may be large losses of sodium potassium and water through the kidneys.

Measurement of urinary excretion of sodium per 24 hours should be carried out. If it is elevated it points to renal loss of sodium.

The laboratory findings are those of a fall in the plasma concentrations of sodium, often potassium and chloride. As most of these patients are anaemic elevation of the haematocrit is unusual, and may not be used as an index of volume depletion.

1.7.1. Treatment of renal loss of sodium
The volume deficiency is estimated from measurements of observed loss, taking into account how much of this has been given over the previous days. The estimated volume deficit is used to replace the calculated sodium loss.

When the urinary volume is increasing, e.g., during recovery from acute renal failure or obstructive uropathy, extra sodium (and potassium) may be needed.

Patients with chronic sodium wasting need extra salt by mouth on a regular basis, 12 g or more being required daily.

1.8. Adrenocortical insufficiency

Mineralocorticoid insufficiency leads to loss of both water and sodium. This occurs in Addison's disease and leads to weight loss, extracellular volume depletion and reduced renal blood flow. Elevated plasma levels of ADH have been reported recently. It is corrected by giving oral salt supplements and an oral mineralocorticoid preparation such as fludrocortisone (Florinef).

Acute adrenal insufficiency (crisis) may occur in patients receiving long-term treatment with corticosteroid, either as replacement therapy after bilateral adrenalectomy or hypophysectomy, or as immunosuppressive therapy. Symptoms usually arise during the stress of acute illness or following operation.

Before the antibiotic era, acute adrenal insufficiency due to haemorrhage into the adrenals was a lethal complication of meningococcal septicaemia (Waterhouse-Friderichsen syndrome).

Symptoms of extreme weakness, lethargy, nausea, vomiting, abdominal pain, fall in blood pressure with shock, or hypothermia in such a patient should arouse suspicion of acute adrenal insufficiency. The biochemical abnormalities are hyponatraemia, hyperkalaemia and hypoglycaemia. The blood urea rises later as the result of reduction in renal blood flow due to hypotension. The plasma cortisol level is usually reduced but may be misleadingly normal. A normal cortisol level is inappropriate for the situation of stress.

1.8.1. Treatment of acute adrenal insufficiency
The treatment is the administration of corticosteroid, giving 250 mg hydrocortisone

6 hourly by intramuscular injection. The dose is gradually reduced in amount and frequency according to response.

1.9. Diabetic keto-acidosis

The osmotic diuresis associated with hyperglycaemia leads to large urinary losses of sodium and water. In severe diabetic keto-acidosis as much as 10% of total body weight may be lost. The high glucose level causes hyperosmolality despite the loss of sodium via the kidneys, and water is withdrawn from cells causing further reduction in extracellular sodium concentration. At a late stage, when there have been very large losses of water, the plasma sodium may become elevated – this is a danger signal of severe hypovolaemia.

The biochemical findings depend upon the severity and duration of the keto-acidosis. Usually, initially, the plasma sodium concentration is reduced, there is an increase in the anion gap (Chapters 1 and 16) as well as an elevated glucose concentration.

It is important to allow for the osmotic effect of glucose when calculating the sodium deficit. For every 10 mmol/l increment in plasma glucose concentration there is a reduction in plasma sodium concentration of approximately 1 to 1.5 mmol/l due to movement of water out of cells and a correction for this needs to be made.

Example:
Plasma glucose 50 mmol/l, sodium 142 mmol/l
Glucose: 50–10 = 40 mmol/l = 10 × 4 mmol/l
Sodium elevation
1.5 × 4 =   6 mmol/l

Therefore, corrected plasma sodium concentration = 142 + 6 = 148 mmol/l.

However at a late stage with very high glucose concentrations hypernatraemia develops because of water loss consequent on the osmotic diuresis.

1.9.1. Treatment of diabetic keto-acidosis

Initial blood samples for urea, electrolytes, pH and blood gases, blood count and blood culture should be taken. When obvious hypovolaemia is present 1 litre of 0.9% saline can be given over the first 30 minutes, otherwise this amount is given over the first hour. A urethral catheter should be inserted if consciousness is disturbed. A central venous manometer to monitor central venous pressure is very useful in elderly patients or those with cardovascular disease. After the first hour the infusion should be given at a rate sufficient to maintain the central venous pressure at 6–10 cm H_2O. One litre may be needed 2 hourly for 4 hours, then 1 litre 4 hourly.

If the pH is below 7.0 or the plasma bicarbonate is below 14 mmol/l sodium bicarbonate is substituted for saline, up to 75 mmol diluted with 5% dextrose provided the plasma potassium concentration is not reduced. If the plasma sodium is elevated above 145 mmol/l the sodium should be given as 0.45% ($\frac{1}{2}$ normal) chloride or as sodium bicarbonate 50 mmol/l (1 mmol/l ml) diluted to 1 litre with 5% dextrose.

The replacement of potassium deficit is an important part of the treatment. The plasma potassium may be low, normal or high despite a large total body deficit of 250–800 mmol.

If the plasma potassium is less than 4.5 mmol/l potassium chloride should be added to the infusion at a concentration of 20–40 mmol/l. When giving potassium the urinary output should be carefully watched lest oliguria continues and the plasma potassium concentration should be monitored every 2–3 hours. Oliguria of itself is *not* a reason for withholding potassium as the low potassium level may be a contributory cause of the oliguria, but in these circumstances careful observation of urinary output, blood pressure and frequent estimations of plasma urea and electrolytes are needed.

Insulin is a necessary part of the treatment of this condition and should be given intravenously or intramuscularly at first. An initial dose of 20 units *soluble* insulin is followed by 6 units per hour according to the level of the blood glucose. The blood glucose should be checked hourly during the first 24 hours to assess the amount of insulin needed. Insulin is adsorbed to glass and plastic tubing but at the rate of infusion indicated adsorption should not be sufficient to prevent effective treatment. The subcutaneous route for insulin administration is not suitable for the management of the acute diabetic with keto-acidosis as absorption is slow (half life of soluble insulin is about 4 hours) and may be uncertain if tissue perfusion is poor. Later doses can be given intramuscularly provided there is no evidence of poor tissue perfusion.

1.10. Paracentesis or acupuncture

The rapid removal of effusions from serous cavities, or acupuncture for the relief of severe oedema, may lead to hypovolaemia, especially if the fluid accumulates rapidly again. If the patient is allowed free intake of water the plasma and therefore extracellular, sodium is reduced, and the ensuing reduction in osmolality leads to water being drawn into cells with the production of cellular overhydration.

This situation is difficult to treat and should be prevented by the cautious use of these techniques.

1.11. Drug-induced sodium loss

Drugs which may cause excessive loss of sodium have been listed in Chapter 4 (Table 8). Diuretics are the most frequent offenders, thiazides, frusemide, ethnacrynic acid and spironolactone may all lead to sodium deficiency.

1.12. Bartter's syndrome

Bartter's syndrome is a genetic disorder in which the primary defect is thought to be in the renal absorption of chloride. Most patients have severe sodium wastage with hyponatraemia, and hypokalaemia. The renal loss of sodium and water leads to volume depletion, secondary hyperaldosteronism and increased renin production with hyperplasia of the juxta-glomerular apparatus. The biochemical abnormality is hyponatraemic hypokalaemic alkalosis.

Sodium loads are excreted very rapidly and intravenous therapy is not indicated except when intercurrent electrolyte disorder occurs. Reports of successful treatment of Bartter's syndrome with indomethacin have appeared.

Reference

1. Alberti KGMM: Diabetic emergencies. Medicine International *1:* 343–345, 1981.

12. Hyponatraemia without sodium loss

When hyponatraemia is present without sodium loss, the plasma sodium is reduced without reduction in total body sodium. The plasma sodium concentration is reduced because of dilution, the causes of dilution being listed in Table 27.

Table 27. Causes of hyponatraemia without sodium loss.

1. Water excess dilutional hyponatraemia
2. Hyponatraemia with hyperlipidaemia
3. Hyponatraemia with hyperproteinaemia
4. Hyponatraemia with hyperglycaemia

1. Dilutional hyponatraemia

This is usually due to continued intake of water in situations in which there is reduced need for water. Intake of water in excess of requirement usually occurs because the decreased need has not been appreciated and normal intake has been continued (Table 28). The hyponatraemia occurring during acute oliguric renal failure, hypotension with reduced urine volume, severe congestive heart failure, cirrhosis of the liver and inappropriate secretion of antidiuretic hormone is due essentially to continued ingestion or administration of water when renal excretion is reduced. In these circumstances both total body water and sodium are increased but the increase in total body water exceeds the increase in total body sodium.

Dilutional hyponatraemia due to irrigation with glycine solution during transurethral resection of the prostate has been mentioned (Chapter 10).

Hyponatraemia may occur in the new-born when the mother has been given dextrose solutions intravenously (as a vehicle for oxytocin). Endogenous secretion of ADH probably increases during labour and synthetic oxytocin in large doses has an antidiuretic effect, contributing to both maternal and foetal hyponatraemia.

1.1. Symptoms and signs of dilutional hyponatraemia

The physical examination may reveal oedema, ascites, elevation of jugular venous pressure, hypertension, pulmonary crepitations. A gain in weight occurs when the

Table 28. Causes of dilutional hyponatraemia due to water excess.

1. Early oliguric acute renal failure with inappropriate water intake
2. During hypotension
3. Severe congestive cardiac failure
4. Cirrhosis of liver
5. Syndrome of inappropriate secretion of antidiuretic hormone
6. Dilutional hyponatraemia of the new-born

cause of hyponatraemia is water excess. Lethargy, apathy, disorientation and muscle cramps are characteristic.

When the onset is rapid, cerebral oedema may develop, with confusion, abnormal behaviour, fits and eventually coma.

Features of the basic disease may also be present.

Reduction in the plasma sodium concentration may be associated with reduction in the haematocrit and plasma osmolality. The potassium level may be low, normal or elevated according to the cause of the basic disturbance. The urinary excretion of sodium is less than 10 mmol/l in cirrhosis and cardiac failure, provided the patient is not taking a diuretic.

1.2. Treatment of dilutional hyponatraemia

Patients in situations where sudden reduction of urine volume may occur need careful observation to avoid fluid overload and dilutional hyponatraemia.

Restriction of water intake is the first line of treatment in most circumstances associated with dilutional hyponatraemia. If an intravenous infusion is being given this should be discontinued. Unless the onset of hyponatraemia has been rapid it is sufficient to reduce the total intake of fluid to 500 to 750 ml daily for a few days. When it has occurred rapidly and the patient is confused or having fits, 5% sodium chloride in small amount is beneficial and leads to increased urinary volume.

If the cause is congestive heart failure a loop diuretic such as frusemide may help excretion of water by increasing renal blood flow without reduction of glomerular filtration rate. It is important to restrict fluid intake at the same time to derive maximum benefit.

2. Hyponatraemia with hyperlipidaemia

In patients with hyperlipidaemia the plasma sodium concentration may be reduced. The increased concentration of lipid occupies volume and displaces water, and reduces the concentration expressed in mmol/l of sodium and other electrolytes. If the excess lipid is removed from the plasma sample, the concentrations of electrolytes become normal.

This form of hyponatraemia does not require treatment.

3. Hyponatraemia with hyperproteinaemia

Increased concentrations of plasma proteins, e.g., due to myeloma, displace water and produce hyponatraemia similarly to hyperlipidaemia.

This form of hyponatraemia does not require treatment.

4. Hyponatraemia with hyperglycaemia

Hyperglycaemia leads to increased loss of sodium by the kidneys, and therefore to true hyponatraemia, but it also causes dilutional hyponatraemia because of osmotic fluid shifts. Each elevation of serum glucose of 10 mmol/l above the normal level decreases the serum sodium concentration by approximately 1.5 mmol/l. The treatment of the hyperglycaemia described (Chapter 11) corrects this abnormality.

13. Sodium excess syndrome

Synonyms: oversalting, extracellular fluid excess

Sodium excess syndrome implies an increase in total exchangeable body sodium. It does not refer specifically to the level of the plasma sodium, which may be low, normal or high. Oedema is usually present.

Increase in total exchangeable body sodium is almost always accompanied by increase in total body water. The clinical manifestation of sodium excess is, therefore, the development of *oedema*. In the ambulant patient the oedema first appears in the feet, increasing in amount towards evening (Fig. 5). At first the oedema may disappear during the night, but appear again as the day goes on. With increasing sodium and water retention the oedema spreads up the lower limbs and is present even in the morning. Later still oedema appears in the sacral area and back, and ascites and pleural effusion (usually but not invariably bilateral) may develop.

In the recumbent bedridden patient not previously oedematous, oedema may develop insiduously because the retained sodium and water are spread over the whole of the large dependent area. It is useful to palpate the back of the thighs in recumbent patients, where the oedema may often be appreciated first (Fig. 6). The whole back, rather than the sacral area only, eventually becomes oedematous.

The characteristic feature of oedema is 'pitting', which is the tendency for the indentation made by gentle pressure by the examiner's thumb or finger to persist. Gentle pressure of 'one finger in one place for one minute' facilitates detection of early oedema.

1. Causes of oedema

The causes of oedema are listed in Table 29.

1.1. Cardiac oedema

When the heart fails as a pump there is a decrease in cardiac output, followed by a decrease in renal blood flow and hence in glomerular filtration rate. The resulting reduction in excretion of sodium and water leads to increased extracellular volume, increased circulating blood volume and increased hydrostatic pressure. Oedema develops in dependent areas because of the increased hydrostatic pressure.

Table 29. Causes of oedema.

1. Cardiac failure
2. Hypoproteinaemia:
    excessive urinary loss
    failure of production
3. Cirrhosis
4. Hormonal oedema:
    Cushing's syndrome
    corticosteroid therapy
    secondary hyperaldosteronism
5. Idiopathic oedema

In some patients with cardiac failure there is increased secretion of aldosterone. This leads to further retention of sodium and increased excretion of potassium. Urinary excretion of sodium is usually less than 10 mmol/l provided that the patient is not taking a diuretic.

There are several theories which attempt to explain the increased secretion of aldosterone in cardiac failure, but it seems probable that the original stimulus is the decreased extracellular fluid volume usually associated with reduced cardiac output. The secretion of aldosterone leads to retention of sodium and water but this of itself is not sufficient to restore the circulation to normal because there is widespread spasm of both small arteries and veins, probably due to sympathetic stimulation. The vascular spasm appears to be the stimulus which leads to continued secretion of aldosterone.

For a fuller discussion of the pathogenesis of cardiac oedema see Davis [1].

1.1.1. *Treatment of cardiac oedema*

Treatment should be directed firstly towards the cause of the cardiac failure (hypertension, anaemia, valvular disease, etc.). The background of cardiac failure is often hypertension, either very prolonged, or very severe, or both. Hypertension, if present, should be brought under control. A diuretic is the first line of treatment. Frusemide 40 mg given intravenously, followed by 40–80 mg orally in the morning, or twice daily if oedema is gross, usually produces a good diuresis. For full benefit from the diuresis it is important to restrict intake of fluids to about 1 litre daily and reduce dietary sodium to 60–80 mmol daily. If the oedema is resistant spironolactone may be given as well as frusemide, to counteract hyperaldosteronism. Later the patient may be treated with a thiazide diuretic on a long-term basis. It should be remembered that thiazide diuretics are much less expensive than frusemide and spironolactone.

Cardiac function may be improved by digitalisation (commence with 0.5 mg digoxin, followed by two doses of 0.25 mg intramuscularly at 6-hour intervals,

0.25 mg daily is given orally thereafter, unless the patient is old, is a child or has impaired renal function when the dosage must be reduced).

1.2. Hypoproteinaemia

In hypoproteinaemia the albumen fraction is reduced, the globulins being normal or slightly raised. However, the increase in globulins is small and is of little significance as their osmotic activity is much less than that of albumen.

Hypoproteinaemia leads to diminution of oncotic pressure within the vascular compartment, with consequent movement of water, followed by sodium, into the extravascular compartment of extracellular fluid. The shift of fluid may be great enough to reduce plasma volume by 20–30%. It seems probable that cardiac output will therefore tend to be reduced and lead to generalised vasoconstriction, but experimental proof of this is lacking.

There is no absolute association of any particular level of the plasma albumen with the occurrence of oedema. Indeed oedema may disappear spontaneously or with therapy with little increase in plasma albumen concentration. A possible explanation may be that the relationship between the volume distribution and plasma protein level is non-linear probably because the tissue fluid is normally held in a tissue gel. Any attempt to draw fluid from the gel leads to negative pressure tending to oppose the removal of more fluid. However, the looseness of the interstitial tissues allows the storage of 5–10 litres of excess fluid without the development of more than minimal increase in interstitial fluid pressure. Put simply, it is easier to accumulate fluid in the interstitial tissue than it is to get rid of it!

Hypoproteinaemia may be due either to excessive urinary loss, gastrointestinal loss, failure of production or starvation.

1.2.1. Hypoproteinaemia due to excessive urinary loss

The 24-hour urinary excretion of protein (mainly albumen) normally does not exceed 200 mg in the male or 500 mg in the female (vaginal secretions contribute to the apparent urinary protein excretion in the female).

An otherwise healthy individual can compensate for considerable urinary loss of protein without developing hypoproteinaemia, and therefore without formation of oedema.

The combination of excessive urinary loss of protein, hypoproteinaemia and oedema is known as the *nephrotic syndrome*.

The main causes of the nephrotic syndrome are given in Table 30.

Increased urinary loss of protein may also occur in hypertension, pyelonephritis, renal tuberculosis and polycystic disease of the kidneys but is rarely great enough to lead to the nephrotic syndrome. Proteinuria rarely exceeds 5 g per 24 hours in these conditions.

Table 30. Causes of the nephrotic syndrome.

1. Primary glomerulonephritis
    minimal change glomerulonephritis
    proliferative glomerulonephritis including
    mesangiocapillary glomerulonephritis
    membranous glomerulonephritis
2. Secondary glomerular diseases

metabolic	diabetes mellitus
immune complex diseases	lupus erythematosis
	vasculitis and polyarteritis
	Henoch-Schöenlein purpura
	sarcoidosis
infections	subacute bacterial endocarditis
	shunt nephritis
	hepatitis B
	malaria
	syphilis
	leprosy
neoplasms	Hodgkin's disease
	lymphoma
	myeloma
	lung, breast, gastrointestinal
	tract, ovary, kidney, cervix
inherited	Alport's syndrome
	Fabry's disease
amyloid	primary
	secondary bronchiectasis
	tuberculosis
	rheumatoid arthritis
	myeloma
toxins	gold, mercury
	penicillamine
	hydrocarbons
	numerous drugs[a]

3. Toxaemia of pregnancy
4. Miscellaneous
    transplant rejection
    poison ivy
    snake venom

[a] See Appendix 6.

1.2.1.1. Treatment of the nephrotic syndrome. If the cause is treatable this should be the first aim in therapy, but a discussion of the treatment of the diseases listed in Table 30 is outside the scope of this book.

Treatment of the oedema itself is the combination of a potent diuretic such as frusemide, with careful restriction of intake of fluid and sodium. If the oedema is severe it is helpful to give the frusemide intravenously (40–160 mg) for the first few days as oedema of the gastrointestinal mucosa may reduce absorption of the drug.

Intravenous infusion of 35 g of salt-poor albumen daily for a few days may help to produce a diuresis if the serum albumen level is 12 mmol/l or less. When the onset of oedema is very rapid hypovolaemia may be severe enough to cause acute renal failure, and albumen infusion helps to prevent this complication.

When a diuresis is obtained it is important to watch the blood pressure and be on guard against the development of hypovolaemia, which may sometimes be severe enough to cause acute renal failure. If hypovolaemia appears imminent it may be averted by a small intravenous infusion of 0.9% saline, and temporary discontinuation of the diuretic therapy.

1.2.2. Hypoproteinaemia due to failure of protein production

Failure of protein production is a comparatively rare cause of hypoproteinaemia. Advanced prolonged liver disease is associated with failure to form albumen.

Reduced production of plasma albumen occurs in the malabsorption syndrome but this is only rarely severe enough to lead to the nephrotic syndrome. However, protein may be lost via the bowel in considerable amounts in ulcerative colitis and in pseudomembranous colitis.

1.3. Cirrhosis

In cirrhosis of the liver, ascites occurs along with oedema. The disorganisation of the architecture of the liver by the cirrhotic process obstructs the portal venous return. This leads to marked congestion of the lymphatics, and the transudation of fluid from the surface lymphatics to form ascites.

Once formed the ascites may lead to decreased circulating blood volume, adrenal stimulation and production of aldosterone.

At a later stage the liver fails to form albumen and this also contributes to oedema and ascites.

Patients with cirrhosis sometimes produce excessive amounts of antidiuretic hormone, leading to water retention and worsening of ascites and oedema.

At a late stage in cirrhosis, cardiac decompensation may develop due to myocardial degeneration perhaps partly from malnutrition (alcoholic cardiomyopathy).

1.4. Hormonal oedema

In Cushing's syndrome and following corticosteroid therapy the oedema is probably due to increased aldosterone secretion leading to sodium and water retention.

Secondary hyperaldosteronism. The reduction in circulating blood volume associated with congestive heart failure, cirrhosis, the nephrotic syndrome and malignant hypertension, stimulates the zona glomerulosa of the adrenals and produces a state of secondary hyperaldosteronism. This causes retention of sodium and water and potassium loss. Secondary hyperaldosteronism, unlike primary hyperaldosteronism (Chapter 14) is associated with severe oedema.

1.5. Idiopathic oedema

This type of oedema occurs in young or relatively young women. They complain of swelling of the face, hands, abdomen and feet. The swelling is often difficult for the observer to detect but they appear to gain several pounds in weight over a day. It is often most marked the week preceding and for a few days following the menses. The patient may appear to be emotionally disturbed. She becomes obsessed with weight and soon discovers that a diuretic leads to loss of fluid and weight. From this it is a short step to the abuse of diuretic drugs to keep to a low (sodium-water-depleted) weight. It is often very difficult to wean the patient off diuretic therapy. I have several times observed women who had taken diuretics to the point of producing hypokalaemia and increase in plasma, urea and creatinine, but who were most reluctant to give them up.

Reference

Davis JO: The pathogenesis of peripheral cardiac oedema. Contributions to Nephrology 21. Bahlmann J, Brod J (eds.). Basel: Karger, 1980, pp 68–74.

14. Hypernatraemia

A plasma sodium concentration of greater than 145 mmol/l usually means that sodium is present in excess of water and other ions.

Hypernatraemia may result from reduction in body water or from increase in body sodium. The causes of hypernatraemia are given in Table 31.

Table 31. Causes of hypernatraemia.

1. Water deprivation (dessication)
2. Increased water loss
   2.1. Diabetes insipidus
   2.2. Excessive renal loss (nephrogenic diabetes insipidus)
   2.3. Infantile hypernatraemia
3. Inappropriate administration of sodium
4. Haemodialysis against concentrated dialysis fluid
5. Hyperaldosteronism
6. Essential hypernatraemia

1. Water deprivation (dessication)

Hypernatraemia associated with water loss has already been described (Chapter 9).

2. Increased water loss

2.1. Diabetes insipidus

Diabetes insipidus (central) with failure of production of antidiuretic hormone, leading to excessive loss of free water is a surprisingly common cause of hyperna-traemia. The commonest cause of this syndrome is head injury, but it may follow intracranial operation, or be associated with supra- or intra-sellar tumours or cysts, meningitis or abscess. In one of my patients diabetes insipidus was due to sarcoid infiltration at the base of the brain. True idiopathic diabetes insipidus is very rare, and hypernatraemia usually does not occur because the thirst mechanism is normal. However, hypernatraemia may develop quickly if a patient with diabetes insipidus becomes unconscious and the attendants are not aware of the need for unusually large volumes of water.

In diabetes insipidus following head trauma or other CNS diseases, the plasma sodium concentration usually exceeds 150 mmol/l and may be as high as 160 mmol/l. The high plasma sodium concentration may persist for weeks even if sodium-free or almost sodium-free fluid (with potassium) is given. Some of the medications given to such patients may contain sodium, and patients with severe head injuries are usually given large doses of corticosteroid to reduce cerebral oedema, which contribute to sodium retention. However, there must be considerable loss of intracellular sodium to account for the continuing urinary loss.

The immediate treatment is the administration of water in the form of 5% dextrose along with potassium chloride appropriate to the urinary loss. The prognosis is related to the likelihood of recovery from the original condition.

2.2. Excessive renal loss of water (nephrogenic diabetes insipidus).

The causes of excessive loss of water through the kidneys have been described already (Chapter 9, Table 23).

2.3. Infantile hypernatraemia

A high serum sodium level sometimes complicates severe gastroenteritis in infants, where the water loss exceeds the sodium loss. This is a serious situation which requires urgent treatment, and there is a high mortality.

The conditions which lead to infantile hypernatraemia are associated with sodium and potassium loss. It is, therefore, appropriate to give some sodium as well as water, as 1/5 normal saline solution, potassium chloride being added at a concentration of 20 mmol/l.

3. Inappropriate administration of sodium

Elevated levels of plasma sodium are more dangerous if they develop rapidly. Rapid elevation of the plasma sodium leads to sudden shrinkage of brain, with rupture of cerebral capillaries and the appearance of petechial haemorrhages. This is most likely to occur if the plasma sodium concentration is raised rapidly to above 160 mmol/l. The mortality is very high, and if survival occurs there may be permanent cerebral damage.

Large amounts of sodium bicarbonate are often given rapidly for correction of acidosis following cardiac arrest, or of acidosis in a patient in respiratory failure on the basis of the pH and blood gas values. The tissue anoxia which accompanies cardiac arrest leads to lactic acidosis (Chapter 16). In both situations plasma sodium is usually normal and sodium given rapidly will raise the plasma sodium concentration well above normal, although with time water will be withdrawn from cells to dilute the sodium concentration.

Sodium bicarbonate is usually given in the concentration of 1 mmol/1ml. Therefore, 100 ml of sodium bicarbonate contains 100 mmol of sodium as well as 100 mmol of bicarbonate. If this is administered *very rapidly* intravenously it could for a very brief time increase the plasma sodium concentration by nearly 28.5 mmol/l.

$$\frac{100 \text{ mmol NaHCO}_3}{\text{plasma volume}} = \frac{100}{3.5} = 28.5 \text{ mmol/l}$$

If the plasma sodium concentration is initially 140 mmol/l (normal), the bolus of 100 mmol of sodium bicarbonate may raise the plasma sodium concentration well above 160 mmol/l. This is well within the danger level for the brain cells. At times considerably larger amounts of sodium bicarbonate may be given rapidly by inexperienced teams treating a patient with cardiac arrest, or by the inexperienced anaesthetist who fails to appreciate that intravenous administration of sodium bicarbonate is not the appropriate therapy for respiratory acidosis. Another hazard of the administration of sodium bicarbonate in these circumstances is acute pulmonary oedema.

If it seems essential to treat acidosis of rapid onset with sodium bicarbonate, considerably less than 100 mmol should be given, and it should *not* be given as a bolus.

Patients requiring intensive care after severe trauma or operation are often given numerous drugs many of which contain sodium, intravenous nutritional solutions and other sodium-containing solutions. They may also be given corticosteroids in high dosage for head injury or other reasons. Renal function may be reduced because of hypotension or frank renal failure may develop. It is not surprising that these patients sometimes develop alarmingly high levels of plasma sodium.

4. Haemodialysis against concentrated dialysis fluid

Haemodialysis against very concentrated dialysis fluid has occasionally occurred because of faulty dialysis equipment. Mulligan et al. [1] reported a patient who developed massive haemolysis with a serum sodium concentration of 177 mmol/l following accidental dialysis against concentrated dialysis fluid. The patient became unconscious for two days after which he made a partial recovery. Over a month he became apathetic with very little spontaneous movement, with evidence increasing cerebral atrophy on CT scans.

5. Hyperaldosteronism

Increased secretion of aldosterone is the normal response to reduction in circulating blood volume, leading to sodium retention by the kidneys, with a modest rise in plasma concentration. In primary hyperaldosteronism, aldosterone is secreted autonomously by the adrenals. This may be due to an adenoma of the adrenal cortex (*Conn's syndrome*) or to bilateral adrenal hyperplasia. This causes chronic retention of sodium and water, with increase in circulating blood volume and extracellular volume. Oedema is *not* a feature of primary aldosteronism (unlike secondary hyperaldosteronism where oedema is marked, Chapter 13), as the renal tubules 'escape' from the effect of excess mineralocorticoid, limiting retention of sodium to 200–300 mmol.

The biochemical abnormality of primary hyperaldosteronism is hypokalaemic metabolic alkalosis. However, Conn's syndrome is a very rare cause of hypokalaemic alkalosis.

6. Essential hypernatraemia

A high serum sodium concentration for which no cause can be found is regarded as essential. True essential hypernatraemia must be rare, but may appear to be present for a time before other symptoms and signs of a brain tumour or other space occupying lesion appear.

7. Treatment of hypernatraemia

The treatment of hypernatraemia depends on the cause. If due to deprivation of water this should be given by mouth. Sodium-containing medication should be stopped.

Reference

1. Mulligan I, Parfrey P, Phillips ME, Brown EA, Curtis JR: Acute haemolysis due to concentrated dialysis fluid. Br med J 284: 1151–1152, 1982.

15. Disturbances of potassium metabolism

Potassium is the main intracellular cation. It is present in muscle cell water at a concentration of about 102 mmol/l. The normal concentration of potassium in extracellular fluid, including plasma, is much lower, varying between 3.5 and 5.0 mmol/l.

The total body potassium amounts to about 3600 mmol, 300–500 mmol being fixed in bone and dense connective tissue, 3000–3500 mmol being within cells and only 60–100 mmol being in extracellular fluid including plasma. The plasma potassium concentration (kalaemia) therefore, gives little information about total exchangeable body potassium. A low, normal or high plasma potassium may be present with a low or normal total exchangeable body potassium. An increase in total exchangeable body potassium does not occur.

Intracellular potassium concentration is not measured in clinical laboratories, and the state of total exchangeable body potassium has to be assessed from the clinical history.

Artefactual elevation in plasma potassium concentration is quite common, e.g., if the blood is haemolysed by shaking the specimen too vigorously, if many bubbles are introduced during withdrawal of the sample, or if the specimen is left at room temperature without separation of cells from plasma (potassium diffuses out of cells). A high plasma potassium level which is not in keeping with the clinical situation should be checked.

1. Potassium and neuromuscular transmission

Changes in plasma potassium concentration are very important because of the part played by potassium in the physiology of muscle contraction. Muscle contraction is initiated by the release of acetyl choline at the neuromuscular junction. The contraction stimulus is conducted along the muscle fibre because of the potential difference produced across the cell membrane by the concentration gradient between potassium within and without the cell. There is a potential difference of 90 millivolts between the inner and outer surfaces of muscle cell membrane. When the muscle is stimulated, potassium moves out of the cell, thus reducing the potential difference (depolarizing) and causing the stimulus to spread along the muscle fibre. A persistent increase or decrease in polarization, due to changes in

112

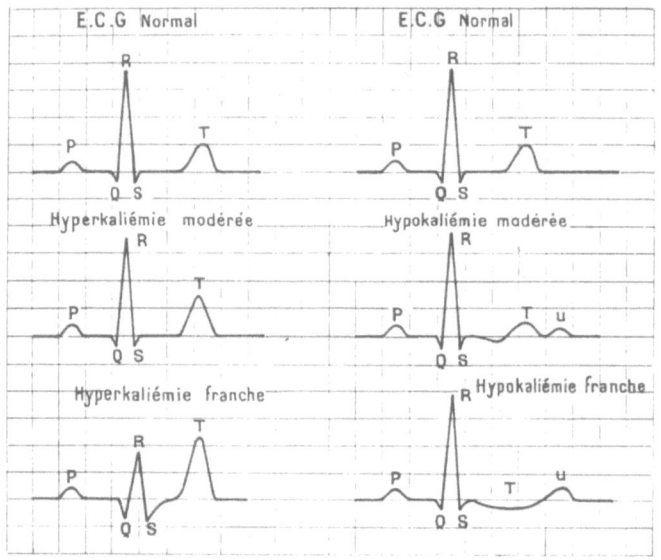

Fig. 12. Schematic representation of the principal electrocardiographic abnormalities associated with variations in the serum potassium concentrations. Diagram reproduced by courtsey of Baillière (Paris) from Équilibre Hydro-électrolytique Normal et Pathologique, G. Richet, R. Ardaillou, C. Arniel, M. Paillard et A. Kanfer (eds.), 1979, p. 144.

extracellular potassium concentration, can block the spread of the stimulus and may cause muscle weakness or paralysis. It follows that either high or low levels of potassium in plasma can cause muscle weakness or paralysis, affecting myocardium, smooth muscle and striated muscle.

Neuromuscular disturbances in the myocardium associated with abnormal concentrations of plasma potassium are reflected in the ECG, and these changes may be present before other evidence of potassium abnormality appears. There is, however, no direct relationship between the presence or degree of muscle weakness and the plasma potassium concentration.

A diagrammatic representation of potassium-associated abnormalities in the ECG is shown in Fig. 12.

1.1. Hyperkalaemia

The ECG changes associated with hyperkalaemia do not appear constantly at any definite elevated level and occasionally the ECG may be normal with a serum potassium concentration of as high as 8.3 mmol/l. With moderate elevation the T waves increase in amplitude and later become peaked (Fig. 13). The PR interval becomes prolonged, the P wave disappears and there is progressive widening of the QRS complex. The rhythm may be regular or irregular and the rate slow or rapid. The presence of high-peaked T waves alone is not diagnostic of hyperkalaemia.

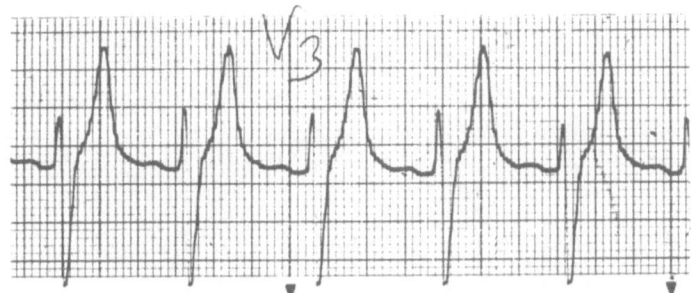

Fig. 13 Electrocardiographic appearances in hyperkalaemia.

The cardiac effects of hyperkalaemia are potentiated by acidosis, hypocalcaemia and hyponatraemia.

1.2. Hypokalaemia

This is associated with lowering and broadening of the T wave, and slight prolongation of the QT interval. With very low plasma potassium levels there is a low broad T wave with the appearance of a U wave, later the T wave becomes depressed and the U wave increases in size, and the QRS interval is prolonged (Fig. 14). Arrythmias including sinus bradycardia, a-v block, paroxysmal atrial tachycardia may occur.

Hypokalaemia is particularly dangerous in patients receiving digitalis, as arrythmias due to digitalis toxicity may be precipitated or made worse.

2. Potassium disturbances and renal function

2.1. Hypokalaemia and renal function

Hypokalaemia may be the result of abnormal renal function and of itself produces profound abnormalities of renal function.

In the presence of hypokalaemia the kidney is incapable of correcting electrolyte disturbances. There is a decreased ability to concentrate urine normally, leading to polyuria. When severe potassium deficiency is present the osmolality of urine decreases to about that of serum (isosthenuria), the low osmolality persisting when fluids are withheld or given. Acidosis cannot be corrected because a sufficiently acid urine cannot be excreted, and in the presence of alkalosis the urine remains acid.

Renal impairment, with increase in serum creatinine and urea, sometimes occurs, particularly when the hypokalaemia is due to gastrointestinal loss of potassium. Deficiency of water and sodium are also present and probably also play a part in the impairment of renal function, which disappears when the electrolyte disturbances

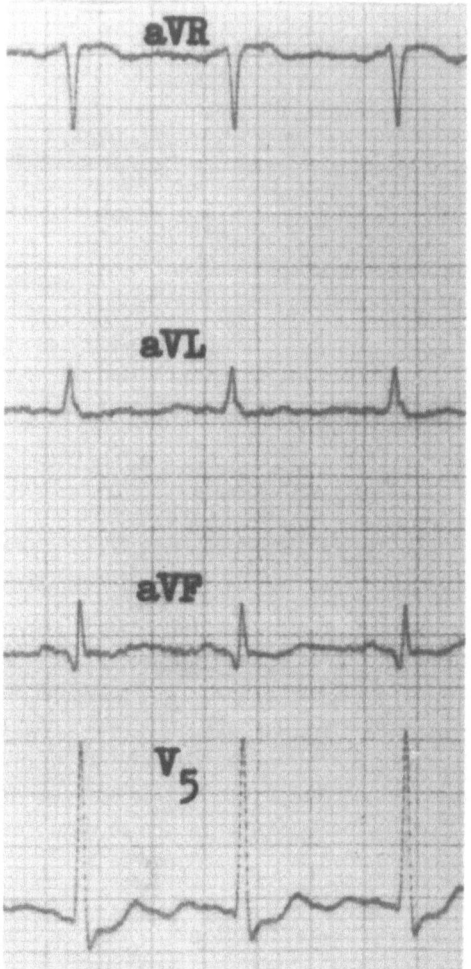

Fig. 14. Electrocardiographic appearances in hypokalaemia. Courtsey of Dr N.P.S. Campbell.

are corrected. Long standing hypokalaemia may be associated with tubulo-interstitial nephritis and proteinuria, usually less than 1.0 g per 24 hours and consisting mainly of globulin rather than albumen.

2.2. *Hyperkalaemia and renal function*

Elevation of plasma potassium concentration is characteristic of acute renal failure and of some types of advanced chronic renal failure. The serum potassium may remain normal in chronic renal failure until the glomerular filtration rate falls below 10 ml/min but may be elevated with a filtration rate well above this level if marked acidosis or excessive catabolism are present, or with actively progressing nephritis.

Hyperkalaemia of itself does not alter renal function.

3. Potassium and acid/base status

Acidosis causes a shift of potassium from cells into extracellular fluid. Therefore, in an acidotic subject an intracellular deficiency of potassium may be present despite a normal or even high serum potassium concentration.

Acidosis and hypokalaemia may occur together when both potassium and bicarbonate are lost, e.g., diarrhoea.

Alkalosis causes a shift of potassium from extracellular fluid into cells. Therefore, in an alkalotic subject the serum potassium may be low without loss of potassium.

Hypokalaemia may thus be associated with metabolic acidosis or alkalosis. Hypokalaemic alkalosis is particularly common in situations where there is loss of H^+ as well as potassium, e.g., vomiting/aspiration; via the kidney due to diuretic therapy, in primary and secondary hyperaldosteronism.

Potassium loss itself causes alkalosis. When potassium is lost from cells, sodium and H^+ move into cells to replace the potassium, in the proportion of 2 sodium ions and one H^+ for every 3 potassium ions. There is, therefore, loss of H ion from extracellular fluid. Potassium loss reduces the number of potassium ions in the renal tubules available for exchange for sodium ions. Hydrogen ions are excreted instead of potassium ions, again leading to metabolic alkalosis. The urine is acid, in spite of alkalosis, a characteristic of metabolic alkalosis due to potassium loss.

4. External potassium balance

Under normal circumstances the potassium contained in the diet amounts to about 75 mmol/l per day. The potassium comes mainly from meat, fruit and fruit juices and beverages, the potassium content of instant coffee being particularly high. About 70 mmol of potassium is excreted in the urine per 24 hours, and about 5 mmol in faeces.

Under abnormal circumstances of excessive tissue breakdown intracellular potassium is lost into extracellular fluid and can lead rapidly to hyperkalaemia, e.g., severe trauma especially with crushing of muscles, large haematoma, severe infection, massive blood transfusion. Patients with severe trauma sometimes develop high output renal failure with massive renal losses of potassium.

5. Hypokalaemia

Hypokalaemia may be due to deficient intake, loss from the gastrointestinal tract or via the kidneys. Loss of potassium via the kidneys may be due to intrinsic renal disease or to the action of hormones or drugs (Table 32).

Table 32. Causes of hypokalaemia.

---

1. Deficient intake
2. Loss of gastric juice
3. Loss of lower intestinal fluids
    3.1. Diarrhoea
    3.2 Abuse of laxatives, enemas
    3.3. Fistulae
    3.4. Tumours
        3.4.1. Gastrinoma
        3.4.2. Villous adenoma
        3.4.3. VIPoma
        3.4.4. Medullary carcinoma of thyroid
    3.5. Ureterosignoidostomy
4. Renal loss
    4.1. Diuretic phase of acute renal failure
    4.2. Following relief of urinary obstruction
    4.3. Pyelonephritis
    4.4. Analgesic nephropathy
    4.5. Drugs
        4.5.1. Diuretics
        4.5.2. Liquorice
        4.5.3. Carbenoxolone
    4.6. Hyperaldosteronism
        4.6.1. Primary (Conn's syndrome)
        4.6.2. Secondary
    4.7. Cushing's syndrome
    4.8. Bartter's syndrome
    4.9. Renal tubular acidosis
5. Familial periodic paralysis

5.1. Deficient intake

Deficient intake of potassium occurs during starvation as in the prisoner on hunger strike already described (Chapter 4). It is more commonly due to insufficient potassium being given to patients requiring intravenous therapy for prolonged periods.

5.2. Loss of gastric juice

Vomiting/aspiration, especially when due to pyloric obstruction, can lead to severe potassium loss with metabolic alkalosis because of loss of H^+. The loss of potassium in gastric juice (15 mmol/l) is less important than potassium loss via the kidneys as metabolic alkalosis stimulates secretion of potassium into the distal renal tubules.

5.3. Loss of lower intestinal fluids

Diarrhoea from any cause leads to potassium loss. Abuse of laxatives (which is often secret) is surprisingly common. Fistulae leading to loss of intestinal fluid or bile may cause serious potassium loss. Some tumours cause diarrhoea but these are rare. They include gastrinoma (Zollinger-Ellison syndrome), non-beta islet cell tumour of pancreas (VIPoma) and medullary cell carcinoma of thyroid. The Zollinger-Ellison syndrome is associated with tumours of G cells, usually in the pancreas. They may be single or multiple and about 60% are malignant. Very large amounts of gastrin are secreted leading to very severe hyperchlorhydria. Severe diarrhoea occurs in part due to ulceration of stomach and intestine and in part due to the low pH inhibiting pancreatic lipase, leading to steatorrhoea. Adenomata of other glands including parathyroid, adrenal, pituitary and thyroid (multiple endocrine adenopathy), are often present. VIPoma is a very rare tumour, secreting large amounts of vasoactive intestinal peptide (VIP), a hormone which increases intestinal motility leading to very profuse diarrhoea. It is associated with achlorhydria and often hypercalcaemia. It is sometimes referred to as the Werner-Morrison syndrome or the WDHA syndrome (Watery Diarrhoea, Hypokalaemia and Achlorhydria).

Marked hypokalaemia is usually present with the hyperchloraemic acidosis associated with ureterosigmoidostomy (Chapter 4).

5.4. Renal loss of potassium

Excessive loss of potassium is common during the diuretic phase of recovery from acute renal failure, and following the relief of urinary obstruction.

Pyelonephritis and analgesic nephropathy may cause renal potassium loss. The association of hypokalaemia with considerable impairment of renal function is suggestive of analgesic nephropathy. Patients who consume large quantities of analgesics may also abuse laxatives and Finn [1] has suggested that hypokalaemia caused by laxative abuse may potentiate the nephrotoxicity of analgesic drugs. Drugs commonly cause excessive renal loss of potassium. Diuretics, especially thiazides, chlorthalidone, xipamide, frusemide and ethnacrynic acid, cause considerable loss of potassium as well as sodium. This may be severe if the patient is taking a sodium-restricted diet, when potassium is excreted along with chloride instead of sodium. Liquorice and carbenoxolone, a liquorice derivative, given for treatment of peptic ulceration both cause significant potassium loss. The active principle of liquorice is glycyrrhinic acid which is structurally and chemically similar to aldosterone.

Hyperaldosteronism leads to renal loss of potassium and hypokalaemia is a characteristic feature of primary hyperaldosteronism (Conn's syndrome). Hypokalaemia may be present in Cushing's syndrome. Bartter's syndrome is another, but very rare cause of hypokalaemia (Chapter 11).

Renal potassium wasting occurs in renal tubular acidosis, and is thought to be an indirect consequence of the impairment of acidification rather than a primary disturbance of potassium transport, as the urinary potassium excretion diminishes when the acidosis is treated. In most patients with renal tubular acidosis potassium supplements are not required when the acidosis is treated with alkali and dietary intake of potassium is normal.

Hypokalaemia is often present in patients with cirrhosis. The use of diuretics, hyperaldosteronism and magnesium deficiency contribute to the hypokalaemia.

5.5. Familial periodic paralysis

In patients subject to familial periodic paralysis, attacks of paresis can occur spontaneously or be precipitated by a large carbohydrate meal or by drugs such as insulin, dextrose, corticotrophin, adrenaline, which reduce the serum potassium concentration. The attacks may occur when the serum potassium is at low normal concentration, e.g., 3.5 mmol/l. The total exchangeable body potassium is normal but lowered muscle potassium concentration has been shown to be present between attacks.

5.6. Symptoms and signs of hypokalaemia

Most of the symptoms and signs of hypokalaemia are non-specific and can occur in seriously ill patients who do not have hypokalaemia.

Thirst, nausea, vomiting, constipation, abdominal distension and paralytic ileus may occur in hypokalaemia but have many other causes.

When the plasma potassium falls below 2.5 mmol/l, muscle weakness may be present and there may be diminished or absent tendon reflexes. Paraesthesiae or pain in muscles may occur. The muscle weakness is most marked in the legs and paresis of the quadriceps may prevent walking. The diaphragm becomes paralysed before the intercostal muscles.

The ECG changes of hypokalaemia have been described already.

Muscle weakness may be the only symptom of chronic potassium loss. Abnormal signs may be absent and even the ECG may be normal. On the other hand polyuria, nocturia and thirst may occur.

5.7. Investigation of hypokalaemia

Very often the clinical history gives important clues as to the origin of hypokalaemia and information on the drugs the patient has been taking may be particularly helpful.

When the plasma potassium is low, the urinary excretion of potassium is usually low also, usually being less than 10 mmol/24 hours. The urinary excretion of greater quantities of potassium is inappropriate in these circumstances, and suggest either renal pathology or renal response to aldosterone as the cause of the hypokalaemia. However, in hypokalaemia associated with gastric loss potassium continues to be lost in the urine despite the low plasma level.

The blood pH, and plasma bicarbonate should be measured.

An intravenous pyelogram may be helpful and may show pyelonephritic scarring or scars left by sloughing of papillae suggesting analgesic nephropathy.

When the diagnosis has not been reached after the above investigations, the possibility of hyperaldosteronism may be considered and plasma aldosterone and plasma renin activity measured.

5.8. Treatment of hypokalaemia

As the plasma potassium concentration does not accord with body exchangeable potassium, the potassium deficiency cannot be quantitated. The only guide to the amount of potassium needed is the clinical situation in which the deficiency has arisen. The deficiency may vary from 250 mmol to 800 mmol or even more. As there is no clear information to the amount needed it is safest to correct the deficiency gradually over several days, or even weeks. Fortunately administration of a small amount of potassium leads to clinical improvement.

The intravenous administration of potassium has been described in Chapter 8.

Chronic potassium deficiency can usually be treated by the oral route. Potassium chloride can be given as a mixture flavoured with syrup of orange. Commercial preparations include effervescent tablets (Sando-K 12 mmol K/tablet; Kloref 7 mmol/tablet) and slow release tablets (Slow K, K Contin and Leo K, all containing 8 mmol/tablet). Intestinal ulceration, haemorrhage and stricture have been reported after administration of Slow K but these complications must be rare as this preparation is widely used. Citrate preparations such as Katorin are more suitable when hypokalaemia is associated with acidosis.

Care is necessary when giving sodium and calcium to patients with hypokalaemia as both exaggerate the neuromuscular abnormalities.

6. Hyperkalaemia

As has been stated already, increase in total body potassium does not occur and hyperkalaemia is due to shift of potassium from cells to extracellular fluid, or to administration of too much potassium.

Hyperkalaemia leads to muscle weakness and paresis. While this affects all muscles, the most important effect is on the heart.

120

Table 33. Causes of hyperkalaemia.

---

1. Acute renal failure
2. Chronic renal failure
3. Acidosis
4. Massive transfusion of stored blood
5. Tissue necrosis, haematoma
6. Drugs
7. Adrenocortical insufficiency (Addison's disease)
8. Hyporeninaemic hypoaldosteronism

Artefactual elevation of the plasma potassium has been mentioned already. Causes of hyperkalaemia are given in Table 33.

6.1. Acute renal failure

This is characteristically associated with elevation of plasma potassium concentration. When the cause of the acute renal failure is severe trauma with tissue necrosis, hyperkalaemia is often rapid in onset. It is particularly severe and rapid when a limb has been crushed ('crush syndrome') and an attempt has been made to conserve doubtfully viable tissue. Muscle necrosis in severe status epilepticus or following coma with prolonged recumbency on a hard surface, produces a similar 'crush' type of renal failure with severe hyperkalaemia. Severe infection may complicate acute renal failure and increase the problem. The hyperkalaemia is due to failure of urinary excretion combined with release of potassium from necrotic cells.

6.2. Chronic renal failure

Hyperkalaemia occurs in many patients with advanced chronic renal failure. Some patients with chronic pyelonephritis, and most with analgesic nephropathy, excrete abnormally large amounts of potassium and even at a very late stage do not develop hyperkalaemia. In most patients with chronic renal failure the serum potassium concentration does not become elevated until the creatinine clearance falls below 10 ml/min unless there is excessive catabolism or severe acidosis. In occasional patients, hyperkalaemia becomes a problem well before renal function falls to this level, even in the absence of hypercatabolism and without very marked acidosis, particularly in patients with declining renal function due to proliferative glomerulonephritis or interstitial nephritis.

6.3. Acidosis

The serum potassium moves from cells into extracellular fluid in acidosis. Rarely this can lead to sudden fatal hyperkalaemia. However it is *not* rare to find hypokalaemia in association with acidosis, e.g., when the acidosis is due to diarrhoeal loss of bicarbonate and potassium, or following ureterosigmoidostomy.

6.4. Massive transfusion of stored blood

The free potassium content of stored blood increases with time of storage. When large transfusions are given following severe trauma, a considerable amount of potassium is given.

A soldier who was accidentally sprayed with bullets from a machine gun sustained rupture of his right kidney and extensive laceration of the liver. By the time I first saw him 36 hours later because of a plasma potassium concentration of 8 mmol/l and acute renal failure he had received 58 units of blood. His right kidney and a considerable portion of the liver had been removed and an abdominal pack was staunching haemorrhage from a large hole in the liver which could not be closed. After 15 haemodialyses he recovered and eventually returned to the army.

6.5. Tissue necrosis, haematoma

Release of potassium from necrotic cells or a large haematoma may be great enough to cause hyperkalaemia, especially if some degree of renal impairment is also present. Anti-neoplastic drugs may cause hyperkalaemia in the same way. (Chapter 4)

6.6. Drugs

The role of drugs in causing hyperkalaemia has been mentioned already. Injudicious intravenous therapy with potassium salts may be expected to cause hyperkalaemia. However, in my experience failure to give sufficient potassium intravenously when it is needed is a much more common error.

The administration of potassium salts by mouth to a patient with chronic renal failure sometimes leads to hyperkalaemia. An episode of vomiting or diarrhoea may cause hypokalaemia in such a patient, which is then treated with oral potassium. The patient may be sent home with instructions to continue the treatment. Once fully repleted again potassium rapidly accumulates, and severe hyperkalaemia may develop. One such patient returned to hospital after a few days complaining that he could not walk. His plasma potassium was 9.0 mmol/l but he too survived, with dialysis treatment and after a renal transplant has returned to full fitness. Administration of potassium-sparing diuretics (spironolactone) to patients with impaired renal function may cause hyperkalaemia.

6.7. Adrenocortical insufficiency

Reduction in secretion of aldosterone in Addison's disease leads to reduced urinary excretion of potassium. Addison's disease itself is rare and severe hyperkalaemia is a rare complication of this rare disease.

6.8. Hyporeninaemic hypoaldosteronism

Damage to the juxta-glomerular apparatus may occur in patients with diabetes mellitus or interstitial nephritis, leading to reduction in renin and aldosterone secretion. The reduction in urinary excretion of potassium may lead to hyperkalaemia. Negroes seem particularly prone to develop this complication of diabetes.

6.9. Treatment of hyperkalaemia

Emergency treatment of hyperkalaemia with intravenous therapy is indicated when the plasma potassium is over 7.0 mmol/l. Bicarbonate, glucose and insulin all cause potassium to move from extracellular fluid into cells. Glucose and insulin (100 ml 25% dextrose given intravenously, followed by 10 units of soluble insulin intravenously) is sufficient when the potassium is less then 8.0 mmol/l. For higher levels bicarbonate, glucose and insulin should be given (75 mmol sodium bicarbonate, 50 ml 50% dextrose, diluted with 5% dextrose to 300–500 ml, given intravenously over 2 hours, 10 units of insulin given intravenously 20 minutes after infusion is commenced). Calcium antagonises the action of potassium on neuromuscular conduction and can be given as calcium gluconate (10–20 ml of 10%). This is effective immediately and is the first line of treatment for life-threatening hyperkalaemia. Calcium should not be given if the patient has received digitalis.

It should be remembered that emergency intravenous treatment of hyperkalaemia is effective for about 4–6 hours and after this potassium may be expected to come out of cells and the plasma concentration to rise again.

When hyperkalaemia is associated with acute renal failure, dialysis should be used to remove potassium from the body. Intravenous therapy (as above) provides time for the patient to be moved to a renal unit and preparations to be made for dialysis. Peritoneal dialysis, using potassium free dialysis fluid at first, is usually sufficient to treat hyperkalaemia, if there is no contra-indication to its use. Haemodialysis can be used to remove potassium more rapidly if necessary, or if abdominal injuries prevent the use of the peritoneal cavity. The soldier injured with machine gun bullets required 15 haemodialyses over three weeks, at first every 24–36 hours.

When hyperkalaemia is associated with chronic renal failure, the plasma potassium usually rises less rapidly. Oral or rectal administration of an exchange resin such as Calcium Resonium can be very effective, the dose being 15–30 g one to four times over the 24 hours. Oral administration of 20 g four times in an average adult male can be expected to reduce the plasma potassium concentration by 1 mmol/1 within 24 hours. Rectal administration of 30 g in 200 ml of water as a retention enema is somewhat less effective. Calcium Resonium given orally causes constipation and a laxative should be given twice daily. Sorbitol syrup (70%) may be given instead of a laxative.

Before Calcium Resonium became available sodium and even aluminium resins were used. The sodium resin released sodium into the large intestine, some of which was absorbed and sometimes contributed to production of congestive heart failure. Calcium is released from Calcium Resonium in exchange for potassium, but absorption of calcium may be helpful as the serum calcium is usually low when renal failure is present.

Dietary restriction of potassium may be needed to prevent recurrence of hyperkalaemia in a patient with chronic renal failure for whom early dialysis is not planned. Restriction of potassium to 50 mmol is fairly easy but is is difficult to reduce potassium intake to less than 40 mmol (about equivalent to 3 g potassium chloride) without making the diet unpalatable.

Reference

1. Finn R, Wainscott JS: Laxan nephropathy. Lancet 1: 1202, 1975.

16. Metabolic acidosis

Synonyms: base deficit, bicarbonate deficit

A careful consideration of the clinical history and physical findings is essential for the diagnosis of acid/base disturbances. The biochemical evidence is often misleading because of compensatory changes which may persist after correction of the basic abnormality, e.g., respiratory alkalosis with metabolic acidosis.

In metabolic acidosis there is excess or relative excess of hydrogen ion. It may result from failure to excrete hydrogen ion, excessive production of hydrogen ion or from loss of bicarbonate. The pH of the blood falls below 7.38 and in extreme situations may fall as low as 6.9.

The body attempts to compensate for acidosis in two ways. The first mechanism is by increased excretion to CO_2 by the lungs. Acidosis stimulates the respiratory centre causing increased rate and depth of respiraton, reducing P_{CO_2} and, therefore, blood H_2CO_3 (respiratory alkalosis, Chapter 1). This compensation is almost always incomplete and is reduced when chronic lung disease is present. The second compensatory mechanism is by increased retention of bicarbonate by the kidneys. When the acidosis is the result of renal disease, renal compensation is reduced or absent.

The compensatory hyperventilation induced by acidosis may persist after correction of the acidosis long enough to cause respiratory alkalosis. The reason for the persistence of the hyperventilation is not known. It is of clinical importance because after the acidosis has been corrected by infusion of sodium bicarbonate or lactate, the continuing compensatory respiratory alkalosis may cause the pH to continue to rise and the actual bicarbonate to fall. It is, therefore, better to monitor progress by bicarbonate and pH levels than the CO_2 content.

Causes of metabolic acidosis. It is helpful to classify acidosis according to whether or not there is a normal anion gap (Chapter 1).

In both types of acidosis the serum concentration of bicarbonate is reduced. When the anion gap is normal, i.e., less than 16 mmol/l, i.e.

$$(Na + K) - (HCO_3 + Cl) \text{ is less than } 16 \text{ mmol/l}$$

the serum chloride concentration rises to fill the gap caused by the decrease in serum bicarbonate concentration – hyperchloraemic acidosis. When the anion gap is increased, unmeasured anions have increased and fill the gap, and the serum chloride concentration remains normal.

Table 34. Causes of hyperchloraemic acidosis (normal anion gap).

_____

1. Diarrhoea and loss from intestinal fistulae
2. Renal tubular acidosis
   2.1. Genetic, with or without other tubular defects (rare)
   2.2. Medullary cystic kidney (fairly common, with nephrocalcinosis)
   2.3. Pyelonephritis
   2.4. Primary hyperparathyroidism with nephrocalcinosis
   2.5. Vitamin D toxicity with nephrocalcinosis
   2.6. Auto-immune disorders:
        hypergammaglobulinaemia
        Sjögren's syndrome
        primary biliary cirrhosis
        lupoid nephritis
        systemic lupus
        cryoglobulinaemia
   2.7. Hypoaldosteronism
3. Ureterosigmoidostomy with long or obstructed ileal loop conduit
4. Chloride acidosis
5. Dilutional acidosis
6. Drug-induced acidosis
   6.1. Acetazolamide
   6.2. Sulphonamides
   6.3. Vitamin D
   6.4. Amphotericin B
   6.5. Heavy metal poisoning: lead, cadmium

_____

1. Metabolic acidosis with normal anion gap

The causes of metabolic acidosis associated with a normal anion gap (hyperchloraemic acidosis) are listed in Table 34.

1.1. Diarrhoea and loss from intestinal fistulae

When diarrhoea occurs, large amounts of bicarbonate are secreted into the gut and excreted. Water and sodium are also lost from the body.

1.2. Renal tubular acidosis

In renal tubular acidosis deficient reabsorption of bicarbonate occurs, with or without failure of excretion of hydrogen ions.

Glomerular function is usually normal and azotaemia is absent.

In proximal tubular acidosis bicarbonate reabsorption is impaired until there is a marked degree of acidosis when bicarbonate reabsorption becomes complete. To this is added potassium loss by the distal tubules. The acidosis is partly buffered by removal of calcium salts from bone and is also often impaired.

In distal tubular acidosis there is failure of excretion of hydrogen ions, again associated with potassium loss.

While renal tubular acidosis may be classified into proximal and distal types, most patients have mixed defects with some failure of bicarbonate absorption and some reduction in excretion of hydrogen ion.

Renal tubular acidosis may be genetic or acquired.

1.2.1. Genetic renal tubular syndromes
There are a number of genetic syndromes, all of which are rare, in which renal tubular deficiencies are present either singly or in various combinations. Renal tubular acidosis may be present alone and associated with renal stones, or be combined with deficient tubular reabsorption of phosphate, glucose or amino acids.

Renal tubular deficiency of phosphate reabsorption, with or without renal tubular acidosis is the commonest of these syndromes, and causes congenital hypophosphataemic rickets. This congenital form of osteomalacia is often familial, it occurs in both sexes but males are usually more severely affected than females. In Fanconi's syndrome, there are defects of tubular reabsorption of glucose, phosphate and amino acids.

1.2.1.1. Diagnosis of renal tubular acidosis. The degree of acidaemia is very variable, the serum bicarbonate ranging from 20 down to 12 or less mmol/l. It is accompanied by hyperchloraemia and hypokalaemia, and hypophosphataemia is often present.

The pH of the urine is characteristically above 6.0 in acidosis of distal tubular origin. It is also usually high in proximal tubular acidosis but may be lower than 6.0 when the plasma pH is very low and accompanied by a low bicarbonate value, when bicarbonate absorption becomes complete. Reduction in phosphate reabsorption occurs in proximal tubular acidosis.

In both types hypercalciuria is the rule. The high urinary excretion of calcium is due to excretion of calcium as base. The hypercalciuria and hyperphosphaturia with urine of a high pH explains the frequency of nephrocalcinosis in renal tubular acidosis. Nephrocalcinosis is not present in the Fanconi syndrome, despite the high urine pH, hyperphosphaturia and hypercalciuria. The Fanconi syndrome differs from the other syndromes in which nephrocalcinosis is common, in that there is increased excretion of amino acids which may inhibit precipitation of calcium salts by chelation.

The absence of hypercalcaemia excludes hyperparathyroidism as a cause of acidosis and hypercalciuria. Drug causes must be excluded.

A confirmatory test for renal tubular acidosis is the response to an oral load of ammonium chloride (0.1 g/kg body weight, usually 8 g ammonium chloride in capsules). This is given at 08.00 hr after collection of specimens of urine at 06.00 hr and 08.00 hr. The patient should be well hydrated and urine samples are collected each hour for 5 hours. The pH of each sample is measured using a pH meter. If the pH does not fall to 5.4 or below, urinary acidification is impaired. The laboratory must be warned in advance that the test is to be carried out as the urinary pH must be measured without undue delay. The test should not be carried out if the patient is already very acidotic, as it may produce symptoms and is in any case unnecessary (if the urine pH is above 5.5 when severe acidosis is present).

1.2.1.2. Treatment of renal tubular acidosis. The treatment is by oral administration of sodium bicarbonate. The dose required varies with the degree of acidosis from 4 to 12 g daily, divided in 3–4 doses as required. Shohl's solution (90 g sodium citrate and 140 g citric acid made up to 1 litre) has also been used in doses of 50–100 ml daily (15 ml = 1.2 g sodium bicarbonate). Adult patients prefer sodium bicarbonate tablets but Shohl's solution is useful for children.

Osteomalacia (rickets) if present will also require treatment with vitamin D during skeletal growth, although correction of acidosis alone may be sufficient in adults.

Correction of the acidosis seems to be beneficial in preserving renal function in patients with nephrocalcinosis. A patient under my care, has shown no reduction in renal function over a 20-year period, nor has she developed hypertension despite regular ingestion of large amounts of sodium bicarbonate.

1.2.2. Medullary sponge kidney
this is a congenital abnormality in which there is dilatation of the collecting tubules in the renal papillea. It is associated with bilateral small renal calculi or nephrocalcinosis. It is not rare but the diagnosis may be overlooked on the intravenous pyelogram if the observer is unfamiliar with the characteristic X-ray appearances. The papillae are broad and flat, with the dilated (sometimes calculi filled) tubules filled with contrast (Fig. 16).

1.2.3. Pyelonephritis
Although impaired reabsorption of bicarbonate or failure to excrete hydrogen ion may result from pyelonephritic renal tubular damage, this is rarely very severe unless glomerular damage and azotaemia are also present.

1.2.4. Primary hyperparathyroidism with nephrocalcinosis
Nephrocalcinosis is not a common manifestion of primary hyperparathyroidism and it is rare to find associated renal tubular acidosis (two out of a personal series of over 350 cases of primary hyperparathyroidism). Multiple, recurrent, or bilateral calculi are much more common although in some patients the diagnosis is made after a single episode of stone. Although there is experimental and clinical evidence that parathyroid hormone inhibits proximal tubular absorption of bicarbonate it is unusual to find acidosis or significant hyperchloraemia in patients with hyperparathyroidism and renal stone disease.

1.2.5. *Vitamin D intoxication with nephrocalcinosis*

Renal stones or nephrocalcinosis due to vitamin D toxicity were not rare before 1960 but are seldom seen now that potent vitamin D preparations are used with greater care and only on clear indications (Chapter 19). Formerly vitamin D was prescribed for treatment of skin lupus, rheumatoid arthritis and given indefinitely (often without regular checking of the serum calcium concentration) if tetany developed after thyroidectomy.

1.2.6. *Auto-immune disorders*

Renal tubular acidosis has been reported in association with hypergammaglobulinaemia (both idiopathic and familial), Sjögren's syndrome, primary biliary cirrhosis, lupoid hepatitis and systemic lupus erythematosis. I have had two patients with renal stones who had Sjögren's syndrome with renal tubular acidosis and hyperphosphaturia.

1.3. *Ureterosigmoidostomy*

Severe acidosis may follow transplantation of the ureters into the colon or into an excessively long (or obstructed) loop of isolated ileum. This is due to bicarbonate loss and reabsorption of chloride from the urine (Chapter 4). Marked hypokalaemia is often present.

1.4. *Chloride acidosis*

The use of ammonium chloride to test urinary acidification can produce worsening of acidosis if already present. Ammonium chloride was formerly used as a diuretic, and when given for weeks, especially when renal function was impaired, produced symptomatic acidosis.

The acidotic effect of giving large volumes of sodium chloride intravenously, especially to a patient with impaired renal function, has been described in Chapter 8. Other chloride salts behave similarly.

1.5. *Dilutional acidosis*

Infusion of large volumes of isotonic sodium chloride reduces the buffering capacity of the sodium bicarbonate/carbonic acid buffer system by dilution. As carbon dioxide and carbonic acid continue to be produced the ratio of bicarbonate to carbonic acid falls producing metabolic acidosis.

1.6. Drug-induced acidosis

Drugs which may cause acidaemia are listed in Table 34.

Acetazolamide (Diamox) produces acidosis by inhibition of carbonic anhydrase, the enzyme essential for the formation (reversible reaction) of carbonic acid from CO_2 and H_2O. Severe acidosis has been reported following its use in patients with mild renal failure. Sodium, water and calcium are excreted in large amounts and renal stones have followed its prolonged use.

Sulphonamides also inhibit carbonic anhydrase. Vitamin D toxicity as a cause of renal tubular acidosis has been mentioned already.

2. Metabolic acidosis with increased anion gap

In metabolic acidosis with increased anion gap the serum chloride concentration remains normal. The increased anion gap is due to the accumulation of unmeasured anions (Chapter 1).

Example: the patient with methanol poisoning described in Chapter 4.

$$(Na + K) - (HCO_3 + Cl) = \text{anion gap}$$
$$(138 + 4) - (7 + 108) = 27 \, \text{mmol/l}$$

Causes of metabolic acidosis with increased anion gap are listed in Table 35.

Table 35. Metabolic acidosis with increased anion gap.

1. Renal failure
    1.1. Acute
    1.2. Chronic
2. Diabetic keto-acidosis, non-ketotic hyperosmolar coma
3. Lactic acidosis
4. Increased catabolism
    4.1. Starvation
    4.2. Fever and infection
    4.3. Violent exercise
    4.4. Convulsions
    4.5. Thyrotoxicosis
    4.6. Surgery and anaesthesia
5. Drugs
    5.1. Salicylate poisoning
    5.2. Methyl alcohol poisoning
    5.3. Ethyl alcohol poisoning
    5.4. Ethylene glycol (antifreeze)
    5.5. Oxalic acid
    5.6. Boric acid
    5.7. Paraldehyde
    5.8. Penicillin and carbenicillin

2.1. Metabolic acidosis due to renal failure (azotaemia)

In normal health the kidneys excrete hydrogen ions in amounts about equal to the daily production by ingestion and metabolism (Chapter 1).

When renal failure occurs the decreased glomerular filtration rate causes retention of hydrogen ions and organic metabolic acids, sulphate and phosphate. Uric acid, phosphoric and sulphuric acids react with sodium bicarbonate with the production of carbonic acid. The carbonic acid dissociates into water and carbon dioxide which is excreted through the lungs. The loss of bicarbonate also contributes to the metabolic acidosis.

Tubular function is usually impaired to some extent and in some diseases this may be disproportionate to the reduction in glomerular filtration (e.g., interstitial nephritis, analgesic nephropathy). Failure to excrete hydrogen ion as ammonium and titratable acid, and sometimes tubular wasting of bicarbonate, contribute to the metabolic acidosis.

Other abnormalities occur, including disturbed potassium metabolism leading to hyperkalaemia or less frequently hypokalaemia (Chapter 15). Hyperphosphataemia plays a very important role in the metabolic disturbances due to renal failure, and may be present early in the course of chronic renal failure before glomerular filtration is greatly impaired. Hyperphosphataemia leads to reduction in the serum calcium concentration, which in turn stimulates secretion of parathyroid hormone (Chapter 19). The resulting secondary hyperparathyroidism leads to one type of renal osteodystrophy and also may increase the metabolic acidosis.

As renal failure becomes worse sodium cannot be excreted normally and there is a tendency for sodium and water retention, leading to congestive heart failure. On the other hand, some patients excrete excessive amounts of sodium and may become acutely salt depleted if deprived of dietary sodium or if vomiting or diarrhoea develop.

Urinary concentration may become impaired and the patient excretes a large volume of dilute urine, and becomes water depleted easily if water is withheld (Chapter 9). At a late stage failure to excrete water and sodium leads to oedema and heart failure.

An account of the many causes of acute and chronic renal failure and their treatment is outside the scope of this book, but the commoner causes are listed in Tables 36 and 37.

It is important to remember that the acidosis of *acute* renal failure usually cannot be corrected by giving sodium bicarbonate. A deficiency of sodium is not present and infused sodium and water cannot be excreted. Administration of sodium bicarbonate sodium is likely to cause left ventricular failure and pulmonary oedema. Acidosis due to acute renal failure should be treated with peritoneal or haemodialysis when the bicarbonate falls below 12 mmol/l.

In most patients with chronic renal failure a similar situation exists. If hypertension and oedema are present already, sodium must not be given. If both are absent a

Table 36. Causes of acute renal failure.

1. Pre-renal
   1.1. Hypovolaemia
      1.1.1. Blood loss
      1.1.2. Plasma loss
      1.1.3. Extracellular fluid loss (external or internal)
   1.2. Hypotension
      1.2.1. Hypovolaemia
      1.2.2. Cardiogenic shock
      1.2.3. Bacteraemia
   1.3. Occlusion of aorta or renal vessels
2. Renal
   2.1. Acute tubular necrosis, cortical necrosis (pre-renal causes)
   2.2. Haemolysis, myolysis
   2.3. Embolism
   2.4. Interstitial nephritis (drugs)
   2.5. Direct drug toxicity
   2.6. Collagen disease
      2.6.1. Systemic lupus erythematosis
      2.6.2. Scleroderma
   2.7. Vasculitis and polyarteritis (drugs)
   2.8. Glomerular nephritis
      2.8.1. Acute
      2.8.2. Rapidly progressive
   2.9. Pyelonephritis (fulminating acute)
3. Metabolic
   3.1. Hypercalcaemia
   3.2. Hyperuricaemia
   3.3. Myelomatosis
   3.4. Hepatorenal syndrome
4. Post-renal
   4.1. Obstructive uropathy
      4.1.1. Calculus (bilateral or obstructing solitary functioning kidney)
      4.1.2. Retro-peritoneal fibrosis
      4.1.3. Tuberculous stricture
      4.1.4. Malignant disease
      4.1.5. Prostatic obstruction
      4.1.6. Urethral stricture

small oral dose such as 3 g daily may be tried and increased if tolerated. Acidosis due to chronic renal failure develops slowly and is remarkably well tolerated, symptoms usually being absent until the bicarbonate falls to 10 mmol/l. The treatment if required, is by peritoneal dialysis or haemodialysis.

Table 37. Causes of chronic renal failure.

1. Glomerulonephritis
2. Diabetes mellitus
3. Severe (malignant) hypertension
4. Pyelonephritis
  4.1. Recurrent
  4.2. With ureteric reflux
  4.3. Analgesic nephropathy
  4.4. With renal calculi
5. Polycystic kidneys
6. Collagen disease
  6.1. Systemic lupus erythematosis
  6.2. Scleroderma
7. Vasculitis and polyarteritis
8. Renal dysplasia and hypoplasia
9. Hereditary nephritis, Balkan nephritis
10. Lead toxicity

2.2. Diabetic keto-acidosis

The primary abnormality in diabetes mellitus is inability to utilise glucose due to deficient secretion of insulin. There is over-production of glucose by the liver which leads to increased concentration of glucose in extracellular fluid. When the renal threshold for glucose is exceeded, glucose acts as an osmotic diuretic causing excessive loss of water and electrolytes including sodium and potassium. Depletion of sodium, water and potassium may be severe.

In the absence of insulin, fat is mobilised and the fat content of blood increases due to increased breakdown of fat deposits as an alternative energy source to carbohydrate. Excessive formation of ketones (beta-hydroxybutyric acid and aceto-acetic acid) leads to the 'unmeasured anion' acidosis. While some of the aceto-acetic acid is metabolised to acetone, other ketones react with sodium bicarbonate, resulting in production of carbon dioxide (excreted by the lungs), decrease in bicarbonate/carbonic acid ratio and further metabolic acidosis.

Failure to metabolise pyruric acid to carbon dioxide may be present in diabetic keto-acidosis and lead to accumulation of lactic acid.

As with any type of acidosis compensatory respiratory alkalosis may occur and may persist for some time after the metabolic acidosis has been corrected.

2.2.1. Treatment of diabetic keto-acidosis

The treatment of diabetic keto-acidosis has been described in Chapter 11.

2.3. Lactic acidosis

Under normal circumstances glycogen in muscle and liver is converted into glucose which is metabolised to pyruvic acid and eventually to carbon dioxide via the Kreb cycle, provided adequate amounts of oxygen are available. Lactic acid is normally produced only in very small amounts. When the tissues are poorly supplied with oxygen, pyruvic acid cannot be metabolised and lactic acid production is greatly increased.

Lactic acidosis often develops rapidly and may be associated with cyanosis. Causes of lactic acidosis are shown in Table 38.

Table 38. Causes of lactic acidosis.

1. Hypoxaemia
    1.1. Shock
    1.2. Cardiac arrest
    1.3. Left ventricular failure
    1.4. Respiratory failure with hypoxaemia
    1.5. Severe anaemia
    1.6. Carbon monoxide poisoning
    1.7. Generalised fits
2. Metabolic acidosis
3. Diabetes mellitus
4. Acute leukaemia
5. Type 1 glycogen storage disease
6. Drugs
    6.1. Ethanol
    6.2. Phenformin
    6.3. Iron intoxication
    6.4. Isoniziad overdose

2.3.1. Hypoxaemia
Any situation in which tissue oxygenation is deficient leads to rapid accumulation of lactic acid. Lactic acidosis therefore occurs in conditions of shock with profound hypotension, during cardiac arrest, in respiratory failure, and left ventricular failure. Lactic acidosis may also be associated with severe anaemia, carbon monoxide poisoning, and generalised fits.

2.3.2. Metabolic acidosis
When marked acidosis develops, inhibition of enzymes leads to accumulation of lactic acid.

2.3.3. Diabetes mellitus
Diabetic keto-acidosis may be associated with lactic acidosis.

2.3.4. Acute leukaemia
There is increased production of lactic acid in acute leukaemia. Infiltration of the

liver by leukaemic cells may impair liver function, and sludging of cells in small vessels may cause tissue anoxia and increase the lactic acidosis.

2.3.5. *Type I glycogen storage disease*
Deficiency of glucose-6-phosphatase leads to failure of formation of glucose from glycogen and accumulation of lactate and pyruvate.

2.3.6. *Drugs*
Ethanol poisoning is associated with increased lactic acid production. Phenformin was formerly used for treatment of diabetes mellitus but has been withdrawn.

2.4. *Increased catabolism*

Increased catabolism leads to increased production of acidic products of metabolism. This may result from starvation or loss of appetite, or the increased catabolism associated with fever, infection, violent exercise, convulsions, surgery and anaesthesia, or thyrotoxicosis.

Metabolism of proteins yields amino acids, phosphoric, sulphuric and uric acids. Fat is broken down into ketone and fatty acids. Carbohydrate metabolism yields lactic and pyruvic acids.

The provision of adequate nutrition for all seriously ill patients is clearly of great importance to prevent these metabolic consequences of the wasting of body tissues.

2.5. *Drugs*

Amongst the drugs which may cause metabolic acidosis salicylate is of particular importance.

2.5.1. *Salicylate poisoning*
Salicylate poisoning is usually due to ingestion of aspirin (acetylsalicylic acid). Salicylate is the active substance in oil of wintergreen (methyl salicylate), salol (phenyl salicylate) and is also available as salicylic acid and sodium salicylate.

Salicylate poisoning is common in small children because 'infant aspirin' comes as raspberry or orange-flavoured tablets.

In adults toxic symptoms may develop because of excessive dosage but may also appear with normal therapeutic dosage if renal function is impaired, or in elderly patients.

Salicylate produces a mixed acid/base disturbance. The immediate effect is stimulation of the respiratory centre, producing hyperventilation and loss of CO_2 leading to respiratory alkalosis. Later it causes depletion of liver glycogen with accumulation of lactic and pyruvic acids. Acute renal failure may develop and increase the acidosis.

2.5.1.1. Symptoms and signs of salicylate toxicity. Tinnitus, vertigo, hearing loss, blurring of vision are early symptoms. The hyperventilation may lead to tetany from alkalosis, the patient complaining of numbness and tingling of the hands and feet or around the mouth. Gastrointestinal symptoms include nausea, loss of appetite and vomiting. Fever, sweating and flushing are common and there may be cyanosis.

As well as hyperventilation there may be excitement, mental confusion, delirium and later lethargy declining into coma and death.

Oliguria is common and proteinuria and haematuria are usually present. Glyco-suria and a diabetic state may occur.

The symptoms and signs of toxicity are not closely related to the amount ingested but are usually present when the blood salicylate level is greater than 30 mg/100 ml. Salicylate can be detected in the urine by adding ferric chloride (10%) to boiling urine when a deep purple colour develops.

2.5.1.2. Treatment of salicylate poisoning. Salicylate poisoning is a medical emergency which carries a high mortality. A stomach wash-out should be given or vomiting induced by ipecacuanha to remove any tablets remaining in the stomach. Recovery of tablets may occasionally confirm the diagnosis before the blood level will be available. Later activated charcoal can be given to absorb salicylate still present in the gut and prevent further absorption into the blood.

Forced alkaline diuresis is indicated (Chapter 8), provided urine is being produced.

If there is reason to believe that a high blood level (over 70 mg/100 ml) is likely the patient should be transferred to a unit able to provide haemodialysis or haemoperfusion, which readily removes salicylate.

2.5.2. Methyl alcohol poisoning

Profound acidosis due to the production of formic acid is characteristic of methyl alcohol poisoning. Blindness is a very common complication.

2.5.3. Ethyl alcohol poisoning

The acidosis is due to production of lactic acid.

2.5.4. Ethylene glycol (antifreeze) poisoning

Ethylene glycol poisoning is usually accidental as in a patient admitted recently to our Unit after taking two mouthfuls of antifreeze from a Coca Cola bottle in the pocket of a car (a common cause of accidental poisoning, particularly in childhood, is the practice of storing poisonous liquids in Coca Cola or lemonade bottles).

Some years ago there was a small epidemic of ethylene glycol poisoning as the result of ingesting antifreeze for 'kicks'. The immediate effect is excitement and confusion with coarse jerking tremors.

Ethylene glycol is broken down into oxalic acid and other organic acids. Oxalic acid crystals are deposited in the kidneys, severe metabolic acidosis and acute renal failure develop. The mortality is high.

Ethylene glycol poisoning should be treated by haemodialysis or haemoperfusion.

2.5.5. Oxalic acid poisoning
Oxalic acid poisoning is rare but similar to ethylene glycol poisoning.

2.5.6. Boric acid poisoning
Boric acid poisoning is usually accidental due to children drinking boric acid solution stored in a soft drink bottle. It can also occur by absorption of boric acid applied as solution or powder to a large area denuded of skin. Deaths have occurred from lavage of body cavities and boric acid is no longer recommended for this purpose.

As well as causing severe acidosis, boric acid poisoning causes vomitus and diarrhoea of blue-green colouration, an erythematous rash, profound shock, sometimes meningeal irritation or convulsions, and coma. Renal failure with oliguria or anuria occurs. The fatal dose in adults is 15–20 g, in children 3–6 g.

2.5.7. Paraldehyde
Very large doses of paraldehyde cause prolonged unconsciousness with respiratory depression and acidosis. There may be an erythematous rash and pulmonary oedema may occur. Kidney function may be impaired. Impaired liver function may increase susceptibility to paraldehyde as it is a liver toxin which may produce toxic hepatitis.

2.5.8. Penicillin and carbenicillin.
These antibiotics behave as unmeasured anions.

3. Symptoms and signs of acidosis

The body tolerates acidosis remarkably well, in contrast to the poor tolerance of changes in osmolality. Mild metabolic acidosis is usually asymptomatic. If the onset has been fairly rapid symptoms begin to appear when the serum bicarbonate concentration falls to 16–18 mmol/l. When acidosis develops very slowly, as in chronic renal disease, symptoms are often absent until the bicarbonate falls to 10 mmol/l or even lower.

The patient may complain of weakness, nausea, vomiting and upper abdominal pain, all of which are non-specific and may be attributed to other reasons. When acidosis is more severe, the patient complains of breathlessness.

The complaint of breathlessness is due to the characteristic deep respirations, usually at a rapid rate (Kussmaul breathing), but sometimes the respiratory rate is not increased. When acidosis is extreme, there may be respiratory depression instead of Kussmaul breathing.

4. Treatment of metabolic acidosis

The treatment of metabolic acidosis should be directed towards the cause of abnormality, as well as attempting to correct the electrolyte disturbance, e.g., treatment of the diabetic state with insulin as well as replacement of deficiencies of water and electrolytes as already described, haemodialysis or haemoperfusion to remove a drug causing metabolic acidosis, or for the acidosis due to acute renal failure.

When acidosis is due to bicarbonate loss from the gastrointestinal tract or via the kidneys intravenous sodium bicarbonate or sodium lactate may be given as described in Chapter 8. Sodium lactate is metabolised to carbonic acid by the liver, which then reacts with the sodium to form bicarbonate. Sodium bicarbonate should be given in situations where lactic acidosis might be expected to develop, e.g., hypoxaemia, or when liver function is impaired.

It should be remembered that potassium loss often accompanies loss of bicarbonate from the gastrointestinal tract. It is very important to give potassium also as correction of the acidosis will increase the hypokalaemia by causing potassium ions to move into cells.

17. Metabolic alkalosis

Synonyms: base deficit, bicarbonate deficit

Metabolic alkalosis is due to loss of hydrogen ion from the body, or to gain in bicarbonate ion. In both situations the bicarbonate/carbonic acid ratio increases leading to a rise in pH.

Compensation occurs in two ways. Alkalaemia depresses the respiratory centre causing shallow breathing, with retention of CO_2, reducing the bicarbonate/carbonic acid ratio towards normal. The respiratory compensation for metabolic alkalosis is less efficient than for metabolic acidosis.

The kidneys attempt to compensate by reduction in excretion of hydrogen ion, chloride and ammonium, and by increased excretion of bicarbonate.

Loss of hydrogen ion may occur from the gastrointestinal tract, from the kidney or via the skin. Net gain in bicarbonate may be the result of oral or intravenous administration of alkalinising salts or of over-compensation for lactic or ketogenic acidosis.

1. Causes of metabolic alkalosis

Causes of metabolic alkalosis are shown in Table 39.

Table 39. Causes of metabolic alkalosis.

---

1. Loss of H^+ via gastrointestinal tract
    1.1. Vomiting/aspiration
    1.2. Congenital chloride diarrhoea
    1.3. Villous adenoma of colon
2. Renal loss of H^+
    2.1. Diuretics
    2.2. Chronic respiratory acidosis
    2.3. Hypercalcaemia
    2.4. Hyperaldosteronism
    2.5. Liquorice, carbenoxolone
    2.6. Cushing's syndrome
    2.7. Bartter's syndrome
    2.8. High renin secretion states
3. Skin loss of H^+
4. Potassium depletion
5. Net gain of bicarbonate

1.1. Loss of H^+ via gastrointestinal tract

1.1.1. Vomiting/aspiration
In the parietal cells of the stomach, carbonic anhydrase forms carbonic acid from carbon dioxide and water. The hydrogen ions pass into the stomach lumen and the bicarbonate enters the blood stream. The gastric fluid lost by vomiting and aspiration contains hydrogen, chloride and potassium. The bicarbonate released into the circulation increases the bicarbonate/carbonic acid ratio, with increase in pH. The hypochloraemic hypokalaemic alkalosis of vomiting/aspiration has been described (Chapter 11).

1.1.2. Congenital chloride diarrhoea
Chloride diarrhoea is a rare syndrome due to a congenital defect of reabsorption of chloride affecting both small and large intestine. The loss of chloride is greater than the plasma concentration and this combined with severe potassium loss leads to metabolic alkalosis.

1.1.3. Villous adenoma of the colon
Villous adenoma of the colon is a rare tumour which may become malignant. It produces diarrhoea containing large amounts of sodium, potassium and chloride. Hypokalaemic alkalosis is due to the loss of chloride and potassium.

1.2. Renal loss of H^+

1.2.1. Diuretic therapy
Diuretics which act mainly on the ascending loop of Henle, including thiazides, frusemide and ethnacrynic acid increase excretion of sodium, potassium and chloride proportionately more than bicarbonate. This is enhanced by sodium chloride restriction. The alkalosis is usually mild.

1.2.2. Chronic respiratory acidosis
The renal mechanism for compensation for respiratory acidosis leads to increased secretion of H^+ (which is excreted with ammonia) with generation of bicarbonate, increasing the bicarbonate/carbonic acid ratio and therefore increasing pH.

1.2.3. Hypercalcaemia
Hypercalcaemia which is *not* due to hyperparathyroidism occasionally is associated with mild metabolic alkalosis. This may be due to release of buffers during destruction of bone.

1.2.4. Hyperaldosteronism
Increased secretion of aldosterone increases reabsorption of sodium, and excretion

of H^+ and potassium by the distal renal tubules. Bicarbonate is retained leading to alkalosis.

1.2.5. Liquorice, carbenoxolone
The active principle of liquorice (used for the treatment of dyspepsia) is glycyrrihic acid, which is chemically similar to aldosterone. When taken to excess it causes hypokalaemic metabolic alkalosis in the same way as aldosterone.

1.2.6. Cushing's syndrome
ACTH-secreting pituitary tumours and primary adrenal tumour or hyperplasia increase glucocorticoid and corticosteroid secretion, with mild mineralo-corticoid effects similar to aldosterone causing alkalosis.

1.2.7. Bartter's syndrome
The hyponatraemic hypokalaemic alkalosis which occurs in Bartter's syndrome has been described (Chapter 11).

1.2.8. High renin secretion states
Situations leading to high renin secretion, e.g., renin-secreting tumours, accelerated hypertension, renal artery stenosis and oestrogen therapy, and secondary aldostero-ne secretion cause renal loss of hydrogen ion, potassium and chloride, with resultant metabolic alkalosis.

1.3. Skin loss of H^+

Some children with cystic fibrosis develop metabolic alkalosis because of marked loss of chloride in excess of bicarbonate, especially if salt intake is low.

1.4. Potassium depletion

Patients with severe potassium depletion may sometimes develop metabolic alkalo-sis, e.g., the prisoner on hunger strike described in Chapter 4 had a serum CO_2 concentration of 44 mmol/l when the potassium concentration was 1.9 mmol/l and chloride 64 mmol/l. However, in this patient and in most others chloride was also greatly reduced, and it is not certain that potassium deficiency *alone* can cause metabolic alkalosis. Moreover, in some situations marked potassium depletion is accompanied by bicarbonate loss.

1.5. Net gain of bicarbonate

Administration or ingestion of sodium bicarbonate, lactate or acetate (which are metabolised to bicarbonate) leads to metabolic alkalosis. The amount of citrate given with very large blood transfusions may be sufficient to cause metabolic alkalosis. However, it is difficult to produce metabolic alkalosis in a normal individual by bicarbonate loading as the kidney responds by increasing bicarbonate excretion.

The combination of milk and alkali is particularly prone to cause metabolic alkalosis. The calcium content of milk and some antacids are important in the pathogenesis of the renal failure which accompanies milk alkali syndrome (which is very rare).

Recovery from lactic or keto-acidosis treated with sodium bicarbonate may be complicated by metabolic alkalosis because of persistence of compensatory respiratory alkalosis for some time ('overshoot alkalosis'). This may be severe after cardiac arrest when large amounts of sodium bicarbonate are given combined with mechanical overventilation, combined metabolic/respiratory alkalosis.

2. Symptoms and signs of metabolic alkalosis

Metabolic alkalosis has many causes and therefore the clinical symptoms and signs are very diverse.

When metabolic alkalosis is produced by taking large amounts of absorbable alkali for a long time, anorexia, nausea and vomiting may occur. Confusion and mental unreliability may be succeeded by drowsiness and coma. Alkalosis reduces the ionized fraction of serum calcium, and the patient may complain of tetany.

Alkalosis shifts the oxyhaemoglobin curve to the left decreasing O_2 release at tissue level. This leads to muscle irritability, and increased susceptibility to cardiac arrythmias.

Apart from the clinical history, assessment of volume, blood pressure and testing for postural hypotension to assess intravascular volume, are important.

Measurement of urinary chloride concentration can be very helpful to predict whether administration of isotonic sodium chloride will correct the abnormality. When the urinary chloride excretion is low (less than 10 mmol/l) the disorder will respond to sodium chloride infusion (gastric fluid loss, intestinal loss of H^+ and chloride, post-hypercapnia). Urinary excretion of chloride of greater than 15 mmol/l does not generally respond to sodium chloride and is characteristic of the hormonal causes of metabolic alkalosis and of severe potassium depletion. Diuretic therapy is associated with high urinary chloride excretion which becomes low when treatment is abruptly discontinued. Measurement of potassium excretion may be helpful, and the renin-angiotensin system may sometimes need to be investigated.

142

3. Treatment of metabolic alkalosis

The underlying condition should be identified and if possible treated. When the metabolic alkalosis is due to excess absorbable alkali this should be discontinued.

Renal excretion of bicarbonate is facilitated by giving sodium chloride and potassium, e.g., treatment of hypochloraemic alkalosis due to vomiting (Chapter II). It has been claimed that gastric loss alkalosis can be corrected by administration of sodium chloride alone. However, I have had to treat a patient after hypochloraemic alkalosis had persisted despite treatment with isotonic sodium chloride for 10 days. The addition of potassium chloride led to rapid recovery. When potassium has been lost it is sensible to replace it!

Acetazolamide may be useful in patients with alkalosis with volume expansion, and leads to increased excretion of bicarbonate and potassium (which must be replaced).

Other chlorides such as ammonium chloride, hydrochloride acid, arginine hydrochloride are not advised and should not be necessary.

When alkalosis is very marked with blood pH of 7.6 or higher, there is a serious risk of cardiac arrythmia. Rapid reduction of the pH is possible using artificial ventilation adjusted to allow accumulation of CO_2, thereby reducing the blood bicarbonate/carbonic acid ratio.

Haemodialysis can be used to correct alkalosis in a patient with renal failure, but the need for this must be very rare. I have not encountered a patient with alkalosis requiring correction by haemodialysis in nearly 25 years.

18. Respiratory disturbances of acid/base

The respiratory disorders of acid/base are due primarily to either decrease or increase in alveolar ventilation relative to the rate of production of CO_2 by metabolism.

A decrease in ventilation leads to CO_2 retention (hypercapnia) and respiratory acidosis. An increase in ventilation leads to increased CO_2 loss (hypocapnia) and respiratory alkalosis. When either situation arises rapidly, e.g., acute pulmonary oedema, the disturbance is more likely to be severe and to produce symptoms.

The body attempts to correct respiratory acidosis or alkalosis in three ways. The first and most rapid response is by the bicarbonate/carbonic acid buffer systems in extra- and intracellular fluid (Chapter 1).

The second compensatory mechanism is the effect of the pH change on the respiratory centre, tending to alter ventilation in the direction opposite to that which produced the abnormality, i.e., respiratory acidosis is compensated by increased depth and rate of ventilation tending to produce respiratory alkalosis; respiratory alkalosis is compensated by shallow breathing tending to produce respiratory acidosis.

The third compensatory mechanism is by increased renal tubular excretion of hydrogen ion and retention of bicarbonate in respiratory acidosis, or by retention of hydrogen and chloride ions with relative increase in bicarbonate excretion in respiratory alkalosis.

Many patients with respiratory acidosis over-compensate and the pH rises above normal. They will then have a high P_{CO_2}, high standard bicarbonate, positive base excess and pH above 7.46 (metabolic alkalosis).

1. Primary respiratory acidosis

Synonyms: hypercapnia, carbonic acid excess, CO_2 retention.

The production of CO_2 by an adult at rest is 15–20 mol per 24 hours. The CO_2 is transported to the lungs as dissolved CO_2 (7%).

The metabolic CO_2 (15–20 mol daily) must be eliminated by the lungs. The CO_2 combines with water to produce carbonic acid which dissociates to hydrogen ion and bicarbonate

$$CO_2 + H_2O \rightleftharpoons H_2CO_3 \rightleftharpoons H^+ + HCO_3^-$$

Table 40. Causes of respiratory acidosis.

---

1. Inhibition of respiratory centre
   1.1. O_2 administration in chronic hypercapnia
   1.2. Cardiac arrest
   1.3. Drugs
   1.4. CNS tumours, haemorrhage infarcts, infection
2. Muscle and chest wall disorders
   2.1. Muscle weakness
   2.2. Flail chest injury
   2.3. Severe kyphoscoliosis
   2.4. Pneumothorax
   2.5. Pickwickian syndrome
3. Airway obstruction
   3.1. Aspiration
   3.2. Epiglottal and laryngeal oedema
   3.3. Severe bronchoconstriction
4. Alveolar causes
   4.1. Pulmonary oedema
   4.2. Pneumonia
   4.3. Atelactasis
   4.4. Massive pulmonary embolism
   4.5. Inhalation of air with high CO_2 content

Under normal circumstances a rise in P_{CO_2} and H^+ stimulates the respiratory centre resulting in increased ventilation with elimination of CO_2 to maintain the P_{CO_2} between 37 ans 43 mm Hg. Respiratory acidosis can result from any condition which affects the respiratory centre itself, the muscles of respiration and the chest wall, or the alveoli.

1.1. Causes of respiratory acidosis

They are shown in table 40.

The commonest causes of respiratory acidosis are depression of the respiratory centre (drugs, administration of oxygen in chronic respiratory acidosis where the response to P_{CO_2} and pH is diminished) and airway obstruction, especially asthma. The alveolar area is so large that respiratory acidosis does not often result from failure of gas exchange at the alveoli, with the exception of acute pulmonary oedema. Inhalation of air with high CO_2 content (anaesthesia, faulty oxygen tent) may cause acute respiratory acidosis.

1.2. Symptoms and signs of respiratory acidosis

The symptoms and signs of respiratory acidosis depend on the situation in which it arises. The level of P_{CO_2} at which coma develops depends on the rate of onset. Muscle twitching, coarse flapping tremor of hands, flaccid paralysis of limbs, myoclonus, drowsiness or convulsions may precede coma. Tachycardia and a widened pulse pressure are common, followed later by hypertension as cerebral oedema develops.

The depression of the central nervous system in respiratory acidosis is due more to fall in the pH of cerebrospinal fluid than to blood pH. Symptoms of respiratory acidosis are more common and more marked than those of metabolic alkalosis because of the ease with which retained CO_2 diffuses across the blood-brain barrier.

The balance of cation/anion remains normal. The P_{CO_2} is raised and the pH falls. The CO_2 and actual bicarbonate are raised and a base deficit is present. The serum sodium may rise slightly and there is usually a raised potassium concentration. In acute respiratory acidosis during anaesthesia early signs are ECG changes of hyperkalaemia.

In most patients respiratory acidosis is associated with hypoxaemia. The patient, however, may be pink and cyanonis is not usually present.

1.3. Treatment of respiratory acidosis

Treatment of the cause of respiratory acidosis is the prime concern of the anaesthetist and is outside the scope of this book. Intubation and assisted respiration are usually required. If due to drug action, the drug should be withdrawn.

When hyperkalaemia and ventricular fibrillation develop with acute respiratory acidosis, intravenous injection of 50 ml 8.4% sodium bicarbonate may be life-saving.

In the anaesthetised patient the colour may be normal and the first sign of respiratory acidosis may be the onset of ventricular fibrillation. (Ventricular fibrillation may be precipitated also by rapid correction of respiratory acidosis.)

1.4. Carbon dioxide narcosis

This may result from a sudden large increase in P_{CO_2} in a patient with chronic pulmonary disease. Above a P_{CO_2} of about 65 mm Hg the respiratory centre no longer responds to changes in carbon dioxide pressure and hypoxaemia becomes the main stimulus to respiration. When oxygen is given in a concentration great enough to raise arterial oxygen saturation (P_aO_2) this stimulus is diminished and ventilation decreases. This results in accumulation of carbon dioxide and worsening of the respiratory acidosis which may lead to coma and death.

The patient with carbon dioxide narcosis may be mentally disturbed, irritable, depressed or euphoric, hallucinate, later becoming drowsy. Sweating and hypertension are usually present.

2. Primary respiratory alkalosis

Synonyms: hypocapnia, carbonic acid deficit.

Primary respiratory alkalosis results in decreased partial pressure of carbon dioxide in alveolar air due to increased ventilation.

Compensatory (secondary) respiratory alkalosis occurs as a result of metabolic acidosis or respiratory acidosis. Secondary respiratory alkalosis may continue after correction of acidosis.

Respiratory alkalosis most often results from stimulation of the respiratory centre, but stimulation of peripheral chemoreceptors and intrathoracic stretch receptors may also produce it (Table 41).

Table 41. Causes of respiratory alkalosis.

1. Central nervous system causes
   1.1. Psychogenic hyperventilation
   1.2. Drugs especially salicylate
   1.3. Brain stem lesions and encephalitis
2. Peripheral chemoreceptors
   2.1. Hypoxaemia
   2.2. Hypotension
3. Intrathoracic stretch receptors
   3.1. Pneumonia
   3.2. Interstitial pneumonitis
   3.3. Pneumothorax
4. Cause uncertain
   4.1. Cirrhosis
   4.2. Gram negative sepsis

2.1. Causes of respiratory alkalosis

2.1.1. Central nervous system

2.1.1.1. Psychogenic hyperventilation. Hyperventilation occurs in acute anxiety states and in hysteria.

2.1.1.2. Drugs. Hyperventilation with primary respiratory alkalosis due to stimulation of the respiratory centre is the early response to salicylate poisoning. Paraldehyde may produce a similar situation. Alcoholic intoxication in delirium tremens causes respiratory alkalosis.

2.1.1.3. Brain stem lesions and encephalitis may stimulate the respiratory centre.

2.1.2. Peripheral chemoreceptors
In many situations with hypoxaemia or hypotension, chemoreceptors within the peripheral circulation stimulate the respiratory centre.

2.1.3. Intrathroacic stretch receptors
Stretch receptors sensitive to 'stiffening' of the lung, e.g., in pneumonia, interstitial pneumonitis or pneumothorax carry stimuli to the respiratory centre.

2.1.4. Hepatic cirrhosis
Respiratory alkalosis is often present with cirrhosis but the mechanism is unknown. It also occurs in gram negative sepsis but the cause is not understood.

2.2. Symptoms and signs of respiratory alkalosis

Hyperventilation with increase in depth (and tidal volume) is characteristic. The respiratory rate may be normal or increased. If the cause is psychogenic, emotional behaviour may be predominant.

The patient may complain of light-headedness (dizziness), tremulousness, palpitations, tinnitus, tingling and numbness around the mouth, hands and feet (tetany due to reduction in ionized calcium concentration as the pH rises).

There may be signs of tetany (Chvostek's and Trousseau's signs).

Cardiac arrthymias may occur and are serious and life-endangering.

There is an increase in blood pH, with decreased P_{CO_2} and bicarbonate.

2.3. Treatment of respiratory alkalosis

Treatment of the basic disturbance causing the hyperventilation is the only effective treatment. If hypoxaemia is present this must be corrected. The tetany associated with hysterical hyperventilation can be relieved by having the patient breathe into a paper bag. The CO_2 content in the bag rapidly increases and continued rebreathing reduces the alkalosis and leads to increase in ionized calcium concentration.

3. Mixed acid/base disturbances

The compensatory mechanisms for the respiratory disturbances of acid/base are comparatively greater than for metabolic disturbances. Compensatory mechanisms may alter the biochemical parameters of acid/base in mixed directions which can be difficult to disentangle. It is therefore very important to assess the clinical situation

148

Table 42. Simple acid/base disturbance.

	pH	P_{CO_2}	HCO_3
Metabolic acidosis	↓	↓	↓
Metabolic alkalosis	↑	↑	↑
Respiratory acidosis	↓	↑	↑
Respiratory alkalosis	↑	↓	↓

Table reproduced by courtesy of Little Brown (Boston) from 'Renal and Electrolyte Disorders', R W Schrier (ed.), 1980, p 170.

carefully. A mixed acid/base disorder may be suspected from the clinical situation and confirmed by biochemical results.

The metabolic (HCO_3^-) and the respiratory (P_{CO_2}) components of the acid/base equation (Chapter 1) always change in the same direction in simple acid/base disturbances (Table 42).

A knowledge of the quantitative response of the compensatory mechanisms to be expected in simple acid/base disorders is helpful. Values outside the 'rule of thumb' approximation (Table 43) suggest a mixed disorder.

It is useful to remember that in respiratory acidosis the actual bicarbonate is greater than the standard bicarbonate (Chapter 7). In respiratory alklosis the situation is opposite, i.e., actual bicarbonate is lower than the standard bicarbonate.

3.1. *Respiratory acidosis and compensatory metabolic alkalosis*

This can occur in a patient with chronic lung disease who develops congestive heart failure and is treated with diuretics. The changes in pH tend to cancel each other and the pH reflects the net effect remaining about normal. The standard bicarbonate,

Table 43. Rule of thumb for acid/base disorders.

Metabolic acidosis	P_{CO_2} should *fall* by 1.0 to 1.5 × the *fall* in HCO_3^- concentration
Metabolic alkalosis	P_{CO_2} should *rise* by 0.25 to 1.0 × the *rise* in HCO_3^- concentration
Acute respiratory acidosis	Plasma HCO_3^- concentration should *rise* by about 1 mmol/l for each 10 mm Hg increase in P_{CO_2}
Chronic respiratory acidosis	Plasma HCO_3^- concentration should *rise* by about 4 mmol/l for each 10 mm Hg increase in P_{CO_2}
Acute respiratory alkalosis	Plasma HCO_3^- concentration should *fall* by 1–3 mmol/l for each 10 mm Hg decrease in P_{CO_2}
Chronic respiratory alkalosis	Plasma HCO_3^- concentration should *fall* by 2–5 mmol/l for each 10 mm Hg decrease in P_{CO_2}

Table reproduced by courtesy of Little Brown (Boston) from 'Renal and Electrolyte Disorders', R W Schrier (ed.), 1980, p 170.

actual bicarbonate and CO_2 content are high because of the metabolic alkalosis, but the actual bicarbonate is higher than the standard bicarbonate because of the respiratory acidosis.

Example:
>> pH 7.44
>> P_{CO_2} 60 mm Hg
>> CO_2 content 37 mmol/l
>> Standard bicarbonate 32 mmol/l
>> Actual bicarbonate 35 mmol/l
>> Base excess + 9 mmol/l

3.2. Metabolic alkalosis and compensatory respiratory acidosis

The biochemical results are similar to those in Section 3.1. The clinical situation should provide the essential clue to which is the primary disorder.

3.3. Respiratory alkalosis and metabolic acidosis

This type of mixed abnormality occurs in salicylate poisoning. The simultaneous presence of alkalosis and acidosis cancel each other out and the pH remains normal. The respiratory alkalosis is associated with a reduced P_{CO_2}, and the CO_2 content, actual bicarbonate and standard bicarbonate are also reduced. The actual bicarbonate is lower than the standard bicarbonate because of the respiratory alkalosis.

3.4. Respiratory acidosis and metabolic acidosis

These seldom occur together but might be produced in a patient with chronic lung disease and congestive heart failure given ammonium chloride as a diuretic. Both abnormalities produce pH changes in the same direction, resulting in a very low pH. The metabolic acidosis causes a low standard bicarbonate, CO_2 content and actual bicarbonate. The actual bicarbonate will be higher than the standard bicarbonate because of the respiratory acidosis.

3.5. Respiratory alkalosis and metabolic alkalosis

This may follow treatment of metabolic acidosis with excessive amounts of sodium bicarbonate or lactate. The compensatory respiratory alkalosis tends to persist and with the excessive administered bicarbonate leads to high pH, high standard bicarbonate, CO_2 and actual bicarbonate. The actual bicarbonate is lower than the standard bicarbonate because of the metabolic alkalosis.

3.6. Metabolic acidosis and metabolic alkalosis

Metabolic alkalosis and metabolic acidosis do not occur simultaneously but they may occur sequentially. They may be suspected when there is marked increase in the anion gap which is much greater than the decrease in plasma bicarbonate. This might occur in a patient with renal failure (metabolic acidosis) who develops severe vomiting (metabolic alkalosis).

Reference

1. Keahny WD: Pathogenesis and management of respiratory and mixed acid/base disorders. In: Renal and Electrolyte Disorders. Schrier RW (ed.). Boston: Little Brown, 1980, p 170.

19. Calcium and phosphorus

Calcium accounts for about 2.3% of fat-free body weight, 99% being in the skeleton and teeth. It accounts for about 25% of bone (dry, fat-free). Calcium is absorbed from intestinal fluid into plasma, from which it passes into extracellular fluid and bone. There is a constant interchange of calcium, calcium being resorbed from bone into extracellular fluid and plasma, to be excreted in the faeces and urine. The calcium excreted in the faeces is a mixture of calcium unabsorbed from the diet and calcium excreted again into intestinal fluid. Sweat contains small amounts of calcium which are usually ignored in balance studies, but with heavy sweating as much as 8 mg per hour can be lost.

The serum calcium in health is maintained at a remarkably constant level varying from 2.20 to 2.60 mmol/l. Several different methods for measurement of the serum calcium are in use and give slightly different normal ranges. Calcium is present in serum in both diffusible and non-diffusible forms; about 60% is diffusible and nearly all of this is in the ionized state; the small non-ionized fraction of the filterable calcium is mainly bound to citrate. The non-diffusible fraction of the serum calcium is bound mainly to albumen and follows changes in the plasma proteins, being raised in conditions in which there is hyperproteinaemia and reduced in hypoproteinaemia.

Phosphorus accounts for about 1% of body weight, 85% being in the skeleton. The amount present within cells is very small yet very important as it provides for the resynthesis of adenosine triphosphate from adenosine diphosphate, a reaction which provides energy for many enzyme-related systems of metabolism, including glycolysis. Phosphate is present in serum almost entirely as phosphate ions, although usually expressed as phosphorus, the level being remarkably constant between 0.8 and 2 mmol/l in adults. It is about 1 to 1.5 mmol/l higher in small children with actively growing bones. It is probable that a very small fraction of the serum phosphate is bound to protein but that the bond is much more labile than is that of protein-bound calcium. The blood cells contain phosphate and if blood is allowed to stand for some time before the serum is separated from cells, an erroneously high level of serum phosphate will be obtained.

The purpose of precise regulation of serum calcium and phosphorus may be to ensure optimum levels for proper mineralisation of bone without production of calcification of soft tissues. It is the ionized fractions of the serum calcium and phosphate which are concerned in biological activity.

There is no constant relationship between the concentrations of calcium and phosphate in the blood. In hyperparathyroidism they change in opposite directions while in other diseases such as osteomalacia both may be reduced.

The plasma calcium is involved in the maintenance of normal neuromuscular transmission. When it is reduced the neuromuscular excitability is increased so that nerve fibres either respond to stimuli below the normal threshold or send off several impulses in response to a single stimulus of normal strength. Hypocalcaemia also increases the excitability of autonomic ganglion cells. The increased excitability of nerve fibres and ganglion cells is a response to a rapid fall in serum calcium rather than to any arbitrary low level. At very high levels of serum calcium, neuromuscular excitability is reduced.

Calcium ions are necessary for the formation of active thromboplastin, and for the formation of thrombin from thromboplastin, so that blood does not clot in the absence of calcium. The lowest level of serum calcium compatible with life is adequate for clotting, but after massive blood transfusion the large amount of citrate present in the circulation may significantly reduce the ionized calcium and contribute to failure of blood clotting.

Phosphate is freely absorbed from the intestine and is filtered by the glomeruli. About 90% of filtered phosphate is usually resorbed by the renal tubules. The daily excretion varies with the dietary intake.

Elevation of the serum phosphate leads to reduction in the serum calcium, but the reverse does not occur.

Calcium and phosphorus metabolism is controlled mainly by parathyroid hormone and vitamin D and their interactions. Other hormones including calcitonin, thyroxine, growth hormone, oestrogens, androgens, glucagon, insulin, cortisol and vasopressin, are also known to influence calcium and phosphorus metabolism but they seem to play little part in normal homeostasis. They can, however, produce serious derangements of calcium metabolism in disease.

1. Parathyroid hormone

The parathyroid hormone (PTH) is a polypeptide consisting of a chain of 84 amino acids. The sequence of amino acids differs slightly from species to species. The hormone is synthesized by the chief cells of the parathyroid glands as a precusor pre-pro-parathyroid hormone which contains 115 amino acids. This is very rapidly converted to pro-PTH, which contains 90 amino acids. The precursors do not appear in the circulation and PTH is secreted as the 1–84 peptide, which is rapidly broken down in liver and kidneys into smaller fragments most of which appear to be biologically inactive. In normal subjects the concentration of PTH when the serum calcium is normal is less than 0.7 ug/l, using a radio immunoassay to the COOH-terminal. The range is different for assays using an antibody to the N-terminal.

The concentration of calcium in serum appears to be the major factor controlling PTH secretion. Reduction in calcium concentration stimulates and elevation suppresses PTH secretion. A fall of as little as 5% in the serum calcium concentration increases PTH secretion within minutes. Hypercalcaemia suppresses PTH, but incompletely, to a basal rate. The phosphate level appears to have no direct effect on PTH secretion, but as elevation of serum phosphate leads to reduction of serum calcium, it indirectly increases PTH. In acute experiments hypomagnesaemia appears to stimulate secretion of PTH but in prolonged hypomagnesaemia PTH secretion is reduced.

PTH acts on bone and kidney to increase the level of calcium in the serum in response to hypocalcaemia. It stimulates the activity of osteoclasts in bone which mobilise calcium and phosphate from the skeleton. At the same time it reduces the urinary excretion of calcium by increasing reabsorption by the renal tubules. These two actions rapidly increase the serum calcium. It also increases the excretion of phosphate by reducing tubular reabsorption thus preventing an increase in serum phosphate. These actions are preceded by a rapid rise in adenosine 3'5'cyclic monophosphate (cyclic AMP) in serum and urine. PTH increases absorption of calcium from the intestine, but this action may be an indirect one mediated by its action on vitamin D metabolism.

PTH increases the citrate level in blood and most tissues of the body, as well as the urinary citrate. It has been shown that citrate is released from bone following injection of PTH.

It has been reported that the plasma uric acid level is increased in hyperparathyroidism, suggesting that PTH influences urate turnover. This is by no means invariable (personal observation), and many patients with hyperparathyroidism have impaired kidney function which may contribute to the raised uric acid levels.

PTH influences the production of other hormones, possibly in part through elevation of serum calcium. It increases the rate of secretion of calcitonin and stimulates the production of 1,25-hydroxycholecalciferol (see Vitamin D). It has been suggested that it increases the rate of secretion of gastrin but there was no evidence of this in my study of patients with primary hyperparathyroidism.

The parathyroids have been shown to be necessary for buffering an acute acid load in nephrectomised animals. In man hyperparathyroidism may rarely produce renal tubular acidosis which is reversed by removal of the overactive gland.

2. Vitamin D

Vitamin D is present in skin as vitamin D_3 (cholecalciferol) which is produced by the action of ultraviolet light on 7-dehydrocholesterol. Although in temperate climates diet is generally thought to be the main source of vitamin D, it is now recognised that the skin may supply a significant amount even in temperate latitudes. Vitamin D_3 is biologically inactive, but after hydroxylation in the liver and kidney it becomes a very potent calcium- and phosphorus-regulating hormone. The actions of PTH and the active metabolites of vitamin D are very closely interrelated and together are mainly responsible for calcium and phosphorus homeostasis.

Vitamin D is obtained from animal foods, mainly butter, egg yolk and fish liver oil, and is absorbed with fats from the small intestine in the presence of bile salts. In man the action of the ultraviolet light in sunlight converts 7-dehydrocholesterol in the sebum of the sebaceous glands to cholecalciferol (vitamin D_3) which is absorbed into the blood stream. However, in temperate zones most of the daily need for vitamin D is supplied in the diet. Vitamin D_2 (calciferol) is synthesised by irradiation of ergosterol, and it is used as an additive to margarine and is a form of vitamin D commonly used in treatment.

Vitamin D_2 and vitamin D_3 are not biologically active, but both are rapidly transported to the liver, a carrier protein being involved. In liver cells both are converted into 25-hydroxyvitamin D_3 (25-OHD$_3$), the reaction requiring ADP, molecular oxygen and magnesium ions. This is the major circulating form of vitamin D, and it is transported by an α-globulin, which although it transports other metabolites of vitamin D, and vitamin D itself, seems to prefer 25-OHD$_3$. According to DeLuca [1] 25-OHD$_3$ at physiological concentrations does not appear to act directly on any known physiological process and requires further hydroxylation before it can act on intestine, bone and kidney. However, MacIntyre [2] believes that 25-OHD$_3$ has weak biological activity. The further step takes place exclusively in the mitochondria of the kidney cells, where it is converted into 1,25-dihydroxy vitamin D_3 (1,25-(OH)$_2$D$_3$). As far as is known the 1-hydroxylase necessary for this step exists only in the kidney. Nephrectomy in animals prevents the appearance of 1,25-(OH)$_2$D$_3$. Nephrectomy also prevents the intestine and bone from responding to physiological amounts of 25-OHD$_3$, although they respond to administered 1,25-(OH)$_2$D$_3$. This has lead to the conclusion that 1,25-(OH)$_2$D$_3$ is the hormonal form of vitamin D which acts on calcium and phosphorus metabolism. It cannot be detected in the serum of anephric patients maintained by haemodialysis. However, such patients do not all develop osteomalacia even if maintained anephric for as long as six years. This and other evidence suggests that other metabolites of vitamin D must have biological activity.

In normal man some of the circulating 25-OHD$_3$ is metabolised to 24,25-(OH)$_2$D$_3$. This reaction is not prevented by nephrectomy indicating that the 24-hydroxylase must be present in other tissues as well as kidney. It is known that it can also convert 1,25-(OH)$_2$D$_3$ into 24,25-(OH)$_2$D$_3$.

The actions of PTH and vitamin D are closely interrelated so that together they provide a sensitive mechanism for the maintenance of serum calcium at normal level. In response to the stimulus of hypocalcaemia, PTH is released and rapidly, within minutes, releases calcium and phosphate from bone by stimulating osteoclastic activity. The presence of 1,25-(OH)$_2$D$_3$ is necessary for this action to occur and PTH probably acts at bone crystal level with the aid of vitamin D already present.

At the same time, PTH acts on the kidney tubules to increase calcium reabsorption and to decrease phosphate reabsorption. PTH also stimulates the production of further supplies of $1,25\text{-}(OH)_2D_3$ from $25\text{-}OHD_3$ in the kidney. The 1-hydroxylation of vitamin D occurs more slowly and the effect on the absorption of calcium by the jejunum takes hours to appear and hours to die away again. The increased absorption of calcium allows the bone store to be replenished. Thus PTH and vitamin D together allow rapid restoration of the serum calcium level if it falls and also provide for its long-term maintenance. The exact roles of $24,25\text{-}(OH)_2D_3$ and $25,26\text{-}(OH)_2D_3$ have not been defined and it is possible that there are other metabolites of vitamin D yet to be discovered.

It has long been known that vitamin D is necessary for the calcification of osteoid to form mineralised bone and that osteomalacia results from deficiency of vitamin D. Indeed the biological activity of vitamin D metabolites has been assayed by their ability to calcify rachitic rat cartilage. The view that $1,25\text{-}(OH)_2D_3$ is the biologically active form of vitamin D does not fit all the known facts about osteomalacia. Anephric subjects in whom there is no detectable $1,25\text{-}(OH)_2D_3$ may not develop osteomalacia even after long periods of time. Patients on anti-convulsant drugs who develop osteomalacia and some patients with nutritional osteomalacia do not have low levels of $1,25\text{-}(OH)_2D_3$ although they tend to have low levels of $25\text{-}OHD_3$. Low levels of $25\text{-}OHD_3$ occur with osteomalacia due to malabsorption. Therefore the feature common to osteomalacia of varying aetiology seems to be low levels of $25\text{-}OHD_3$ rather than of $1,25\text{-}(OH)_2D_3$.

Muscular weakness is another symptom associated with vitamin D deficiency which rapidly disappears when D_3 or its metabolites are given. The extensor muscles of the thighs are commonly the most severely affected muscle groups so that the patient may have difficulty in rising from a squatting or sitting position or in climbing stairs.

Although osteomalacia, the disease of vitamin D deficiency, is corrected by vitamin D there is no satisfactory evidence that it or its metabolites act directly on the mineralisation of bone. From the evidence available it appears that the curative effect is an indirect one via elevation of serum calcium and phosphate.

3. Vitamin D and the serum phosphate

Vitamin D stimulates the uptake of phosphate from the intestine, and this effect seems to be due to $1,25\text{-}(OH)_2D_3$ as D_3 and $25\text{-}OHD_3$ are effective only in non-nephrectomised animals. However, $1,25\text{-}(OH)_2D_3$ will produce an increase in serum phosphate even when the diet is almost completely lacking in phosphate, showing that it can also withdraw phosphate from bone. Phosphate may play a part in the regulation of $1,25\text{-}(OH)_2D_3$ but the available evidence is inconclusive. In the intact animal calcium depletion stimulates phosphate absorption from the intestine via stimulation of production of $1,25\text{-}(OH)_2D_3$, so that deficiency of either calcium or phosphate stimulates intestinal absorption of both.

Vitamin D metabolites seem to have a dual action on renal phosphate, reducing urinary phosphate excretion when serum phosphate is low, increasing phosphaturia when serum phosphate is elevated.

Hyperphosphataemia leads to reduction in the serum calcium which stimulates PTH production. It is doubtful whether hyperphosphataemia can of itself stimulate PTH secretion.

The serum phosphate level is very important for skeletal health. In some forms of osteomalacia the main abnormality is a low serum phosphate, the serum calcium remaining normal or nearly so. In congenital hypophosphataemic rickets ('vitamin D-resistant rickets') a high renal threshold for tubular reabsorption of phosphate leads to very low levels of serum phosphate. In this type of osteomalacia, mineralisation of bone can be partially restored by raising the serum phosphate either directly by giving phosphate supplements or indirectly by giving vitamin D to increase absorption of phosphate by the intestine.

4. Calcitonin

In man and other mammals calcitonin is secreted by para-follicular or C cells which are derived from the neural crest. In man most of these cells are situated in the thyroid. They may be present in the thymus or the parathyroids and in some species are present in the ultimobranchial bodies.

Like parathyroid hormone, calcitonin is secreted continuously under normal circumstances and secretion is increased in response to hypercalcaemia resulting in reduction of the serum calcium. Secretion appears also to be stimulated by increased levels of plasma magnesium.

Calcitonin inhibits the resorption of bone. Inhibition of bone resorption is most marked in conditions where bone turnover is rapid (e.g., active Paget's disease) and cannot readily be demonstrated in more stable situations. It increases the urinary excretion of both calcium and phosphate by inhibiting tubular reabsorption.

5. Thyroxine

In normal circumstances, thyroxine probably does not take part in calcium homeostasis. However, hypercalcaemia is occasionally present in thyrotoxicosis and hypercalciuria is almost invariable. Increased glomerular filtration occurs in thyrotoxicosis and may contribute to the hypercalciuria.

Thyroxine leads to increased turnover of bone, and some degree of osteoporosis is common in severe thyrotoxicosis. Thyrotoxicosis is sometimes the cause of premenopausal osteoporosis, the thyrotoxicosis sometimes being occult and not clinically obvious.

6. Adrenals

Under normal circumstances cortisol probably has not part in calcium regulation. The serum calcium is sometimes raised in Addison's disease and in one series of 62 cases, eight had hypercalcaemia. Adrenalectomy in dogs is followed by hypercalcaemia and it has been shown that this hypercalcaemia occurs in the absence of the parathyroids. There is no increase in the absorption of calcium, in fact, there is a persistently negative calcium balance during the period when the serum calcium is rising. It is accompanied by an increase in plasma citrate, and this taken together with the above findings, makes it likely that there is increase in resorption of bone.

Patients with Cushing's syndrome may develop osteoporosis, and this is also a not uncommon complication of prolonged treatment with cortisone. Cortisone may induce a negative calcium balance by increasing both faecal and urinary excretion of calcium. In sarcoidosis and in vitamin D intoxication, cortisone reduces raised serum calcium to normal by decreasing calcium absorption with increase in faecal calcium.

7. Growth hormone

Growth hormone appears to affect bone both by the formation of increased collagen and by its effect on vitamin D metabolism. In the rat, hypophysectomy greatly reduces the serum levels of $1,25\text{-}(OH)_2D_3$, which is restored to normal by administration of growth hormone. The increased production of $1,25\text{-}(OH)_2D_3$ caused by secretion of growth hormone provides for the increased absorption of calcium and phosphorus needed for active skeletal growth. Similar changes occur in acromegaly. Parathyroid hyperplasia may be present in acromegaly and may lead to hypercalcaemia.

8. Insulin

Insulin causes phosphate to enter into cells along with glucose. This may indirectly affect serum calcium by stimulation of production of $1,25\text{-}(OH)_2D_3$ by the reduced serum phosphate.

9. Calcium absorption

The absorption of calcium from the diet is incomplete, and varies with the adjustment of the subject to the calcium content of his diet. In an individual adjusted to a high calcium intake, change to a low intake at first results in a negative calcium balance because a large percentage of the dietary calcium is not absorbed. The efficiency of absorption increases as the low intake is continued and the faecal loss falls. The power to adapt in this way may differ in different individuals. A greater proportion of ingested calcium is absorbed in the young, and during pregnancy and lactation. Man can thus remain in calcium balance over a wide range of intake. The minimum requirement for dietary calcium is about 800 mg for adults, and 1.5–2.0 g daily for children and lactating women.

Calcium absorption is in part conditioned by the other items of the diet. High phosphate diets, and those containing excessive amounts of phytate reduce absorption of calcium. Fatty acids in the diet form insoluble soaps and failure of fat absorption leads to decreased calcium absorption. It has been found that calcium absorption from diets deficient in protein is impaired. The calcium in milk is better absorbed than any inorganic or organic salt of calcium (82% of milk calcium absorbed compared with 32% from calcium chloride). Milk calcium is thought to be better absorbed because it is in the form of calcium caesino-phosphate, but in calves it has been shown that lactose increases calcium absorption. Vitamin D is essential for absorption of calcium and PTH also influences it.

The faecal calcium is mainly made up of calcium not absorbed from the diet, but some is actively secreted into the intestine. The *secreted* calcium in faeces amounts to about 70 to 100 mg daily and it is independent of dietary calcium intake. Large intravenous injections of calcium do not appreciably increase faecal excretion of calcium, suggesting that this is not an important route of calcium excretion. It can, however, lead to increase in negative balance as calcium excretion in faeces continues even in starvation, and in severe vitamin D deficiency. The *total* calcium in the faeces amount to about 700–800 mg per 24 hours.

10. Urinary excretion of calcium

Calcium is filtered at the glomerulus but most of the filtered calcium is reabsorbed by the renal tubules. The amount finally excreted in the urine is partly dependent on the dietary calcium intake and to a smaller extent on other items in the diet, and increases with increasing age and skeletal weight. However, in different individuals of similar weight on similar diet there is a wide range of values for urinary calcium and there are various definitions of what constitutes hypercalciuria.

On a normal diet (containing about 1 g of calcium) the urinary calcium excretion per 24 hours seldom exceeds 7.5 mmol in women and 8.5 mmol in men.

When renal function is impaired the urinary excretion of calcium is low. The filtered load of calcium is reduced firstly by reduction in serum ionized calcium due to the increased percentage complexed to citrate and other organic acids, and secondly by the reduced glomerular filtration. Hyperphosphataemia in azotaemia also contributes to reduction in filtered calcium.

11. Hypercalciuria

Increased urinary excretion of calcium is one of the most common abnormalities discovered during investigation of patients with renal stones.

Hypercalciuria may result from increased calcium resorption from bone as in primary hyperparathyroidism, increased intestinal absorption of calcium, or reduced renal tubular calcium reabsorption. The mechanism of absorptive hypercalciuria has not been elucidated but it appears to be independent of vitamin D. The cause of the renal leak of calcium is also not understood but other tubular defects such as impaired concentrating ability, and possibly a leak of magnesium may be present. Some patients experience a urinary infection prior to the onset of stone disease suggesting that hypercalciuria may be acquired.

Increased urinary excretion of calcium occurs in certain diseases (Table 44).

Table 44. Causes of hypercalciuria.

---

1. Hormonal
   1.1. Hyperparathyroidism
   1.2. Thyrotoxicosis
   1.3. Cushing's syndrome, steroid therapy
   1.4. Acromegaly
2. Immobilisation
   2.1. Following fractures
   2.2. Poliomyelitis
   2.3. Paraplegia
   2.4. Tuberculosis of bone
3. Vitamin D intoxication
4. Sarcoidosis
5. Renal tubular acidosis
6. Tumours destroying bone
7. Syndrome of inappropriate secretion of antidiuretic hormone
8. Idiopathic (with renal stones)

11.1. Causes of hypercalciuria

11.1.1. Hormonal causes of hypercalciuria
These have been mentioned already.

11.1.2. Immobilisation
Immobilisation of the skeleton leading to resorption of bone (acute osteoporosis) was formerly a common cause of renal stones, especially in patients with poliomyelitis, tuberculosis affecting bones or joints, or paraplegia. Attention to early mobilisation and high fluid intake has almost eliminated this cause of renal stones.

11.1.3. Vitamin D intoxication

Hypercalciuria occurs at an early stage of vitamin D overdose, before hypercalcaemia and it may lead to formation of stones. This is probably mainly due to increase in filtered load caused by increased calcium absorption and increased bone resorption.

11.1.4. Sarcoidosis

In sarcoidosis there is increased intestinal absorption of calcium, perhaps due to enhanced sensitivity to vitamin D. Hypercalcaemia may occur and hypercalciuria may occasionally lead to stone formation.

11.1.5. Renal tubular acidosis

The hypercalciuria of renal tubular acidosis has been described (Chapter 16).

11.1.6. Tumours eroding bone

Tumours which frequently metastasize to bone include breast, thyroid, lung, hypernephroma, prostate, cervix, ovary. Hypercalcaemia is often present in myelomatosis.

11.1.7. Syndrome of inappropriate secretion of antidiuretic hormone

An increased fractional excretion of calcium has been found in patients with SIADH [4] when the patients are hyponatraemic. The increased calcium clearance appears to be due to the volume expansion. Mild hypocalcaemia and hypercalciuria are common in SIADH.

11.1.8. Idiopathic hypercalciuria with stones

Hypercalciuria associated with renal stones, for which no cause has been found is considered to be idiopathic. It may accompany medullary sponge kidney which is a congenital abnormality (Fig. 15).

11.2. Treatment of hypercalciuria

Treatment for hypercalciuria should be directed at the cause if one is found. Failing this in theory treatment should be based on whether the hypercalciuria is due to hyperabsorption or renal leak, but this is often not practical in the clinical situation. Treatments from absorptive hypercalciuria include:

11.2.1

Moderate *dietary restriction of calcium* (400–600 mg/day).

11.2.2

Cellulose phosphate to block absorption of calcium (5 g three times daily). This,

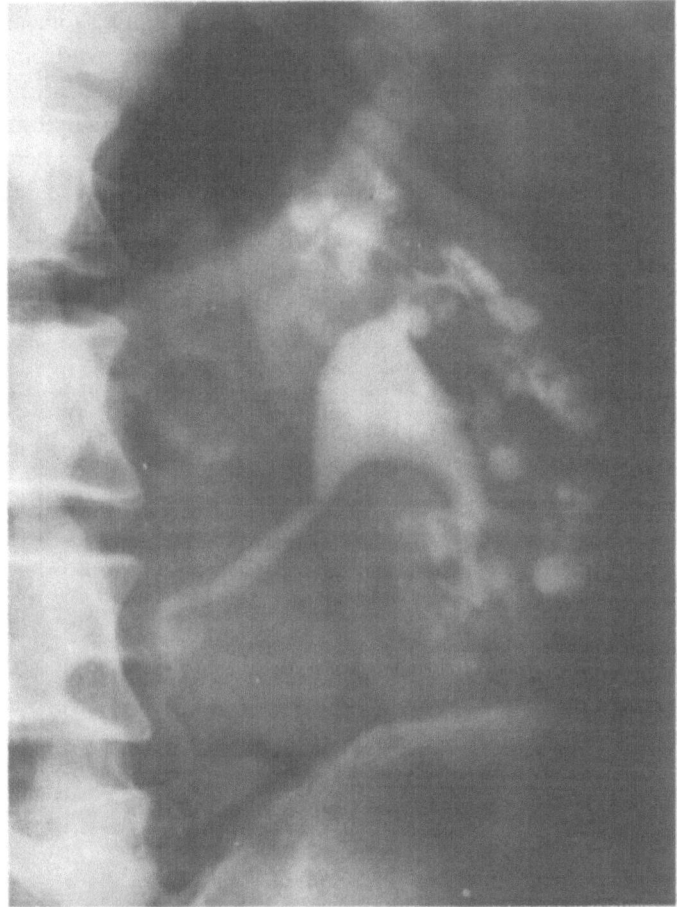

Fig. 15. Medullary sponge kidney with nephrocalcinosis. Note flattened calyces with calcium deposits in dilated collecting tubules.

however, increases urinary excretion of oxalate and phosphate, and reduces urinary magnesium.

11.2.3. Thiazide diuretic

Thiazides reduce urinary calcium excretion by an unknown mechanism. Hydrochlorothiazide 50 mg twice daily, or chlorthalidone 50 mg daily have been used.

Treatment must be life long and patients tend to discontinue treatment. Remission of stone formation has been reported in 70–90% of patients on each of these treatments but other factors including fluid intake may have contributed to the good result.

12. Reduced urinary excretion of calcium

This is of little clinical significance since it does not in itself produce disease, and is usually secondary to other conditions, e.g., hypocalcaemia from any cause, or reduction of glomerular filtration rate, except for the rare syndrome of familial hypocalciuric hypercalcaemia. Symptoms are often absent in family members with hypercalcaemia and the bones are usually radiologically normal although there is an increased prevalence of articular chondrocalcinosis in older patients. There are two important though uncommon clinical associations, acute pancreatitis, and severe neonatal hyperparathyroidism.

13. Hypocalcaemia

The concentration at which reduction in the serum calcium produces symptoms varies with the rapidity of onset and in different individuals. Causes of hypocalcaemia are given in table 45.

Table 45. Causes of hypocalcaemia.

---

1. Hypoparathyroidism
   1.1. Post-operative
   1.2. Idiopathic
2. Malabsorption syndrome
3. Renal failure
4. Nephrotic syndrome
5. Massive blood transfusion
6. Pseudohypoparathyroidism
7. Medullary cell carcinoma of thyroid

13.1. Causes of hypocalcaemia

13.1.1. Hypoparathyroidism
The serum calcium may fall soon after thyroidectomy due to disruption to the blood supply to the parathyroid glands, or following parathyroidectomy (either because too much glandular tissue has been removed, or blood supply has been disrupted). Symptoms are usually present.

13.1.2. Malabsorption syndrome
There are many causes of malabsorption, any of which may lead to hypocalcaemia. Malabsorption of vitamin D as well as calcium is important in the production of hypocalcaemia, as is malabsorption of protein contributing to hypoalbuminaemia. Symptoms may be absent.

The malasorption of calcium is usually associated with other deficiencies. Besides the presence of anaemia (which is not invariably macrocytic) helpful simple screening tests include serum albumen, serum iron and total iron-binding capacity, serum B_{12} and folate, serum carotene. Confirmatory tests include a barium meal with follow-through using flocculent barium, faecal excretion of fat (mean daily excretion of fat in a 3-day collection of faeces should not exceed 5 g), radioactive carbon breathalyser test and intestinal biopsy.

13.1.3. Renal failure

Hypocalcaemia occurs within 24–48 hours of the onset of acute renal failure and is present in chronic renal failure until a late stage when secondary hyperparathyroidism may supervene. Retention of phosphate appears to be the main reason for the fall in serum calcium although calcitonin also becomes elevated. Other suggested explanations for the hypocalcaemia of chronic renal failure are that there is skeletal resistance to the action of PTH, or that vitamin D metabolism may be altered.

Symptoms of hypocalcaemia are only occasionally present.

13.1.4. Nephrotic syndrome

Hypocalcaemia is almost always present in the nephrotic syndrome. This may be due to urinary loss of calcium-binding carrier protein or of vitamin D binding globulin. The plasma $25(OH)_2D_3$ level is usually low in the nephrotic syndrome.

Symptoms of hypocalcaemia are exceptional.

13.1.5. Massive blood transfusion

The citrate contained in massive blood transfusion may be sufficient to cause hypocalcaemia.

13.2. Symptoms and signs of hypocalcaemia

There is no absolute level at which symptoms of hypocalcaemia appear, and a rapid fall from a high level to low normal levels may produce symptoms while a much lower level may be well tolerated if the onset is gradual. The acid/base status is relevant here, acidosis increases the ionized calcium and protects against hypocalcaemic symptoms while alkalosis may be associated with symptoms even when the serum calcium concentration is normal.

The symptoms consist of pins and needles in the extremities, numbness around the mouth and sometimes twitching of the facial muscles. Muscle spasms occur, starting with a feeling of stiffness and going on to a tonic painful contraction which may be described as cramp. This may follow voluntary actions such as writing, holding a steering wheel, etc. The fingers are flexed at the metacarpal-phalangeal joint, and are held tightly bunched together, with the thumb forcibly adducted. The palm is hollowed and the wrist is flexed. When the feet are affected, the toes are flexed under the feet, pressed together with the big toe underneath the others. The posterior muscles of the leg contract and draw the heel upwards. These spasms are known as carpo-pedal spasms. Spasm of the glottis may cause stridor, and spasms of the diaphragm, back or chest muscles have also occurred. Latent tetany may sometimes be demonstrated by the following tests.

13.2.1

Chvostek's sign is elicited by tapping on the facial nerve in front of the ear. A positive sign is twitching of the facial muscles, especially of the upper lip, though occasionally the alae of the nose and eyelids may also twitch.

13.2.2

Trousseau's sign is elicited by raising the blood pressure cuff on the upper arm above the systolic pressure. When positive the hand assumes the position of carpal spasm.

13.2.3

Erb's sign is the demonstration of hyperexcitability of the muscles to electrical stimulation.

13.2.4

Cataracts are common complication of hypoparathyroidism, but may occur in any condition in which there is long continued hypocalcaemia. Atrophic changes may occur in hair, nails, teeth and skin. Monilial infections of the nail beds are relatively common.

13.3. Treatment of hypocalcaemia

Treatment may be required for the relief of tetany. Slow intravenous injection of 10–20 ml 10% calcium gluconate gives immediate relief and also serves to distinguish tetany from other causes of muscle spasm and cramp. Longer term treatment of hypocalcaemia consists of giving vitamin D in some form, the dose depending on the cause, the choice being:

13.3.1. Calciferol (vitamin D₂)

This form of vitamin D does not elevate the serum calcium for about 10 days, but it is cheap and effective. As it is stored in the liver and adipose tissue its effect is cumulative. The dose required may vary from 1.25 mg twice weekly for chronic renal failure to as much as 5 mg daily for idiopathic hypoparathyroidism. The dosage must be controlled by weekly estimation of the serum until a dose is found which maintains the serum calcium at about 2.1–2.2 mmol/l. As the effect is cumulative the aim should be a low normal serum calcium. It is usually possible to manage with estimation of the serum calcium at three month intervals once a suitable dose has been found. As the urinary calcium excretion may be elevated without hypercalcaemia, occasional estimation of the urinary calcium may be helpful.

13.3.2

Dihydrotachysterol (DHT) is a synthetic preparation available only as an oily solution (ATIO) until recently. It is now available as tablets, (Tachyrol), containing 0.2 mg of DHT.

13.3.3

1α-*hydroxyvitamin D₃* is a synthetic analogue of vitamin D marketed as One-Alpha-Leo. The dose is 1 microgram daily, increasing the dose by 1 microgram daily at two weekly intervals until hypercalcaemia appears or the dose of 3–4 micrograms is reached, after which the dose is reduced again. The serum calcium should be measured weekly until the stable dose is established after which it should be measured monthly. It is claimed that hypercalcaemia disappears more rapidly after stopping treatment than with calciferol or dihydrotachysterol. When used for treatment of renal osteodystrophy it is essential to monitor the serum calcium frequently as hypercalcaemia will lead to further deterioration of renal function.

13.3.4. 1,25-dihydroxycholecalciferol

This is thought to be the most active metabolite of vitamin D. It has been used as a research tool in the study of renal osteodystrophy, but in some patients with chronic renal failure it has failed to produce remineralisation. It is not in general therapeutic use.

14. Hypercalcaemia

Hypercalcaemia may lead to a variety of non-specific symptoms or symptoms may be completely absent. It is sometimes associated with bone disease.

Table 46. Causes of hypercalcaemia.

1. With radiological bone disease
   1.1. Secondary carcinomatosis
   1.2. Myeloma
   1.3. Hyperparathyroidism with bone disease
   1.4. Sarcoidosis
   1.5. Acute osteoporosis
2. Without radiological bone disease
   2.1. Hyperparathyroidism
   2.2. Tumours without metastases
   2.3. Vitamin D excess
   2.4. Myeloma
   2.5. Sarcoidosis
   2.6. Thyrotoxicosis
   2.7. Milk alkali syndrome
   2.8. Addison's disease
   2.9. Infantile hypercalcaemia
   2.10. Thiazide-induced
   2.11. Tuberculosis (?)

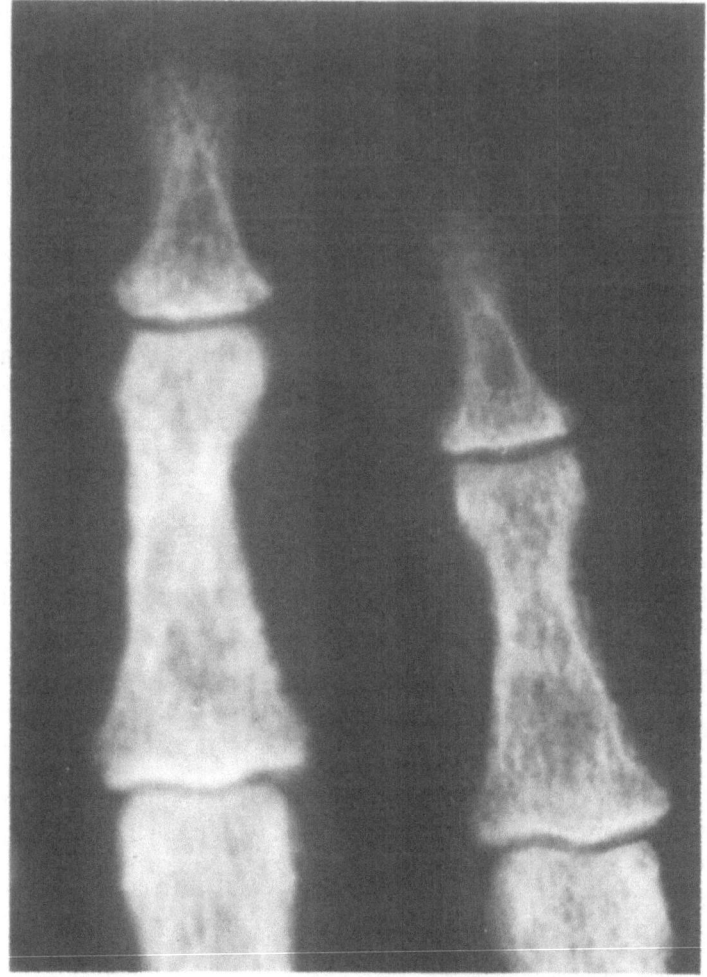

Fig. 16. Primary hyperparathyroidism. Subperiosteal erosions of phalanges.

It is an aid to diagnosis to classify the causes of hypercalcaemia according to whether or not radiological bone changes are present. The causes are given in Table 46 in order of frequency of occurrence.

14.1. Causes of hypercalcaemia

14.1.1. With radiological bone disease

14.1.1.1. Secondary carcinomatosis. Malignant tumours of breast, bronchus, prostate, thyroid and cervix tend to metastasize to bone. Examination of these areas and a chest film are mandatory.

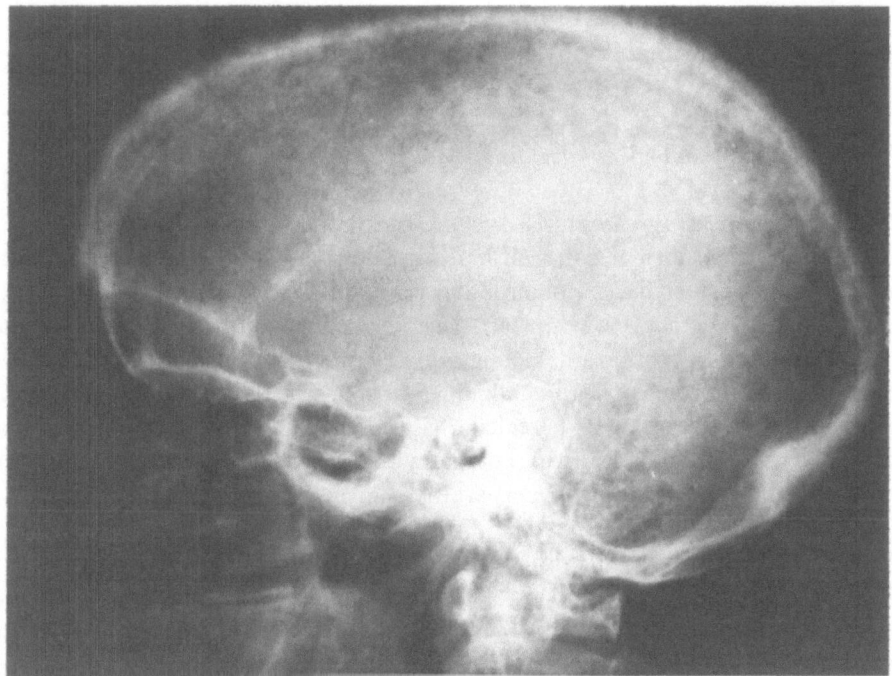

Fig. 17. Primary hyperparathyroidism: granular appearance with subperiosteal erosions of the tables of the skull.

14.1.1.2. Myeloma. Myeloma deposits occur in bone, and in the skull may resemble hyperparathyroidism but hyperparathyroid subperiosteal erosions in phalanges and metacarpals are absent. Hypophosphataemia is absent and the alkaline phosphatase is usually not raised. A raised erythrocyte sedimentation rate (ESR) and myeloma protein in plasma and urine are present.

14.1.1.3. Hyperparathyroidism. The radiological changes of hyperparathyroidism are characteristic and once seen are usually easily distinguished from those of the other causes of hypercalcaemia. All bones are affected and the subperiosteal erosions affecting the fingers occur only in hyperparathyroidism (Fig. 16). The finely granular appearance of the skull is also characteristic (Fig. 17). Moderate to high elevation of the serum alkaline phosphatase accompany hypercalcaemia and hypophosphataemia.

14.1.1.4. Sarcoidosis. The hypercalcaemia of sarcoidosis is thought to be due to excess production and reduced clearance of 1,25-dihydroxycholecalciferol. Small cysts may be present in the carpus but the bones elsewhere are unaffected. X-ray chest and plasma proteins often suggest the diagnosis.

168

14.1.1.5. Acute osteoporosis. Hypercalcaemia may occur in acute osteoporosis in immobilised patients but this is rare.

14.1.2. Without radiological bone disease

14.1.2.1. Hyperparathyroidism. This is the commonest cause of hypercalcaemia with radiologically normal bones. It may be associated with renal stones, mental and emotional disturbances, polyuria and polydipsia, anaemia, or be completely asymptomatic. Non-specific symptoms such as tiredness, poor appetite, constipation are common. Hypophosphataemia (unless renal function is impaired) normal ESR and plasma proteins, normal alkaline phosphatase (unless radiological bone change is present) are usual. Hypercalciuria is present when renal function is normal but is not a useful diagnostic test as it occurs with other types of hypercalcaemia and also with renal stones without hyperparathyroidism.

14.1.2.2. Tumours withour metastases. Certain tumours cause hypercalcaemia in the absence of bone secondary deposits. These include hypernephroma, squamous cell carcinoma of bronchus, and ovarian tumours. This appears to be due to secretion of a PTH-like substance. Hypophosphataemia is usually but not invariably absent and the ESR is usually raised.

14.1.2.3. Vitamin D excess. The history of vitamin D ingestion should provide the essential clue and there should be evidence of the underlying disease for which it was prescribed, e.g., osteomalacia, replacement therapy in hypoparathyroidism, renal osteodystrophy. The serum phosphate may be an unreliable guide as it is low in congenital hypophosphataemic rickets. Hypercalcaemia due to vitamin D excess is reduced to normal by five to ten days' treatment with cortisone acetate (150 mg/day). This cortisone suppression test is both diagnostic and therapeutic.

14.1.2.4. Sarcoidosis. Hypercalcaemia in sarcoidosis has been mentioned already.

14.1.2.5. Sarcoidosis. The abnormalities in plasma proteins, raised ESR and an abnormal chest X-ray (usually present) help to establish the diagnosis. The hypercalcaemia responds to cortisone.

14.1.2.6. Thyrotoxicosis. Hypercalcaemia is rare in thyrotoxicosis although hypercalciuria is very common. The serum phosphate is normal, if reduced co-existing hyperparathyroidism should be considered. Despite the hypercalciuria renal stones hardly ever occur.

14.1.2.7. Milk alkali syndrome. Milk alkali syndrome occurs in patients with peptic ulceration who have taken large amounts of milk and absorbable antacids, especially those containing calcium carbonate. It was formerly though to be quite common but is probably rare. Severe dyspepsia and peptic ulceration occur fairly frequently in primary hyperparathyroidism and many supposed cases of milk alkali syndrome may have been due to hyperparathyroidism. The hypercalcaemia with alkalosis leads to marked impairment of renal function. In the early stages PTH is normal but secondary hyperparathyroidism due to renal failure may lead to a later elevation.

14.1.2.8. Addison's disease. Hypercalcaemia in Addison's disease has been mentioned already.

14.1.2.9. Infantile hypercalcaemia. Infantile hypercalcaemia was first described in 1952 and occurred in artificially fed babies. Failure to thrive, vomiting and constipation were associated with anaemia and moderate impairment of renal function. It was thought to be due to excess vitamin D in infant foods and elimination of vitamin D from the diet led to recovery, though the serum urea sometimes remained elevated. After 1957 the vitamin D content in infant foods was approximately halved, and the disease gradually became rare. Cortisone appeared to be beneficial but less so than in adult vitamin D intoxication.

14.2. Symptoms and signs of hypercalcaemia

Many of the symptoms are non-specific. The patient may feel weak and tired, and the appetite is poor. Nausea and vomiting are common, and in more serious cases there is thirst or polyuria. The urine volume is often increased although this may not be noticed. The patient may go insidiously into renal failure, or this may occur more dramatically when very high levels of serum calcium occur. The patient rapidly becomes dehydrated and oliguric and may die unless promptly treated. Most patients are constipated, and a normochromic anaemia is often present. In milder cases associated with primary hyperparathyroidism, the patient sometimes only recognises the symptoms after recovery of full health following surgical removal of the tumour.

Hypercalcaemia of any cause may lead to impaired renal function. Infusion of calcium into the normal subject depresses the creatinine clearance. In hypercalcaemia deposition of calcium occurs in the kidneys, and although renal function usually improves after treatment some residual impairment of function often remains.

A careful physical examination of the patient with hypercalcaemia may be helpful. The sites of tumours often associated with hypercalcaemia should be examined, i.e., thyroid, breasts, and pelvis.

A scheme for the investigation of hypercalcaemia is shown in Table 47.

The value of the serum phosphorus concentration as a pointer to hyperparathyroid has been mentioned. A low value suggests it and a high value makes it unlikely.

Table 47. Scheme for investigation of hypercalcaemia.

1. Repeat serum calcium to exclude laboratory error
2. Serum phosphate: low favours hyperparathyroidism; high hyperparathyroidism unlikely
3. ESR: usually normal in hyperparathyroidism, usually raised in myeloma and other malignancies
4. Alkaline phosphatase: usually normal in myeloma with bone lesions, normal in hyperparathyroidism without bone disease, raised with bone disease
5. Plasma protein electrophoresis and test urine for Bence-Jones protein: if normal myeloma unlikely but not entirely excluded
6. X-ray chest: tumour, primary or secondary? sarcoid? distal end of clavicles normal?
7. X-ray hands, skull: sarcoid, hyperparathyroidism, myeloma
8. Cortisone suppression test
9. PTH (radioimmunoassay)

The ESR is usually normal in hyperparathyroidism and usually raised in myeloma and other forms of malignant diseases.

The alkaline phosphatase is helpful only when radiological bone changes are present, when it is raised in hyperparathyroidism, usually normal in myeloma. The cortisone suppression test (already described) should be carried out when there is reason to suspect sarcoidosis or vitamin D intoxication, when it is helpful to confirm the diagnosis and is therapeutic. It is not a routine test. Elevation of serum PTH in the presence of normal renal function is diagnostic of hyperparathyroidism but it may be misleading due to technical error (Chapter 7), and the result takes at least a week to arrive by which time the diagnosis has often been reached.

14.3. Treatment of hypercalcaemia

The treatment depends on the cause. The treatment of primary hyperparathyroidism is removal of the overactive gland or glands.

Hypercalcaemia due to other causes and associated with symptoms or with a serum calcium concentration of above 3.0 mmol/l requires treatment.

If the patient seems quite well, renal function is unimpaired, and the serum phosphate is not elevated, oral phosphate is quite effective. It can be useful in elderly patients with primary hyperparathyroidism whose general condition makes surgery inadvisable.

It can be given as Phosphate Sandoz, 2–4 tablets daily. The lower dose should be prescribed at first as oral phosphate may cause diarrhoea.

When the patient is acutely ill and the serum calcium is very high the patient is usually dehydrated and may be oliguric. Rehydration and sodium repletion with 0.9% sodium chloride (about 1 litre every 6 hours) is the first line of treatment and usually leads to improvement in the urinary output. Intravenous frusemide increases calcium excretion.

Buffered sodium phosphate solution may be given intravenously but there is a risk of producing soft tissue calcification and renal damage if the serum calcium is above 3.3 mmol/l.

The use of cortisone to reduce hypercalcaemia due to vitamin D excess and sarcoidosis has been mentioned. Hypercalcaemia due to malignant disease also often responds to steroid therapy. The response in myeloma is less predictable.

Calcitonin given intravenously produces a modest fall in serum calcium and in my experience has been disappointing for severe hypercalcaemia.

Mithramycin, a cytotoxic agent, given intravenously produces a rapid fall in serum calcium but there is a risk of profound hypocalcaemia and it is toxic to the liver and bone marrow.

Peritoneal dialysis or haemodialysis using calcium-free dialysis fluid can be used, when the above measures fail.

15. Hypophosphataemia

Hypophosphataemia may be present when total body phosphorus stores are normal, but in certain circumstances it indicates phosphate deficiency.

Phosphate depletion with a moderately reduced serum phosphate does not produce symptoms and signs. The serum phosphate is moderately reduced in primary hyperparathyroidism and in some patients with renal stones, and in osteomalacia. When the serum phosphate falls below 0.6 mmol/l there is probably a generalised phosphate depletion which is associated with malfunction of most of the body's systems. This situation usually occurs in patients who are already very ill and the symptoms and signs of phosphate depletion are non-specific and easily overlooked, or attributed to other aspects of the illness.

Table 48. Causes of severe hypophosphataemia.

1. Malabsorption due to drugs
2. Burns
3. Parenteral hyperalimentation
4. Re-feeding syndrome
5. Alcohol withdrawal
6. Hyperventilation
7. Diabetic keto-acidosis

15.1. Causes of severe hypophosphataemia

15.1.1. Malabsorption due to drugs
Large doses of aluminium hydroxide, aluminium carbonate or magnesium hydroxide may cause hypophosphataemia when dietary intake of phosphate is low.

15.1.2. Burns
Hypophosphataemia occurs a few days after extensive burns. This may be due to hyperventilation and respiratory alkalosis increasing glycolysis and using up phosphate.

15.1.3. Parenteral hyperalimentation
Many of the solutions for parenteral use are deficient in phosphate, and if phosphate is not provided, severe hypophosphataemia will develop.

15.1.4. Re-feeding syndrome
In re-feeding after starvation hypophosphataemia may develop when calories are provided in normal quantities. This syndrome was described after World War 2 when prisoners developed oedema, ascites and sometimes died when re-fed, especially with carbohydrates.

15.1.5. Alcohol withdrawal
Chronic alcoholics usually eat poorly and are mal-nourished. They often develop ketosis and this may lead to increased urinary excretion of phosphate. Hyperventilation is common and stimulates glycolysis. On re-feeding they may behave similarly to mal-nourished prisoners.

15.1.6. Hyperventilation
When prolonged hyperventilation is present intracellular alkalosis becomes very pronounced because of loss of intracellular CO_2 (which readily diffuses out of cells). The alkalosis increases glycolysis, using up phosphate, which is withdrawn from serum leading to a very low level of serum phosphate.

15.1.7. Diabetic keto-acidosis
The acidosis associated with severe keto-acidosis increases metabolism of intracellular organic phosphates, with release of phosphate which is excreted. The serum and urine phosphate are usually normal or even elevated before treatment of keto-acidosis but falls rapidly when treatment is commenced.

15.2. Symptoms and signs of hypophosphataemia

The symptoms and signs of severe hypophosphataemia are non-specific and are easily attributed to other causes in seriously ill patients. A list of them by body systems is given in Table 49.

15.3. Treatment of hypophosphataemia

Some of the effects of severe hypophosphataemia may be irreversible. Awareness that hypophosphataemia may occur in severely ill patients and timely measures of

Table 49. Effects of phosphate depletion.

System	Effects
CNS	Irritability, increased reflexes, paraesthesiae, confusion, convulsions, coma
CVS	Reduced cardiac contraction, reduced stroke volume
Muscular	Weakness, rhabdomyolysis
Haemopoetic	Reduced life span of RBCs, haemolysis, increased affinity for oxygen leading to tissue anoxia, reduction in phagocytosis and bacteriocidal activity of WBCs, reduced platelet survival, thrombocytopenia
Renal	Reduced excretion of titratable acid, fall in glomerular filtration rate, reduced excretion of phosphate, hypercalcaemia, increased excretion of calcium; metabolic acidosis
Enzymes	Many enzyme activities reduced

prevention are very important. Treatment of the basic clinical situation is critical.

In treating hypophosphataemia there is a risk of producing hyperphosphataemia and soft tissue calcification, especially in lung, kidney, myocardium and blood vessel walls. This is unlikely when giving phosphate orally, unless oliguria and renal failure are present. Milk is a good source of phosphate (1 quart contains 1 g phosphate, 33 mmols) and other nutriments. Phosphate Sandoz, 2–4 tablets daily, is a convenient form of treatment, but should be commenced at the smaller dose as diarrhoea may occur until the intestine becomes tolerant to it, when the dosage can be increased.

Alcoholic patients may require intravenous therapy and this can be given as potassium phosphate (50 mmol/day is usually safe) as potassium depletion is usually also present.

References

1. DeLuca HF: Vitamin D metabolism. Clinical Endocrinol 7, Suppl: 1S–17S, 1977.
2. MacIntyre I: Le rôle du rein dans le metabolisme de la Vitamine D. Actualités Nephrologiques de l'Hôpital Necker. 151–161, 1978.
3. DeLuca HF: Vitamin D metabolism and function. New York: Springer Verlag, 1979.
4. Decaux G, Van Laethen Y, Van Kuyck M, Mackel J: Hypercalciuria in the syndrome of inappropriate secretion of antidiuretic hormone. Mineral Electrolyte Metab 7: 192–196, 1982.

20. Magnesium

Magnesium resembles potassium in being a major intracellular cation and in that there is no direct correlation between serum magnesium concentration and total body magnesium. About 40–50% of the body magnesium is in muscle and considerable amounts are stored in bone. Unlike potassium, insulin does not cause magnesium to shift into cells from extracellular fluid. It resembles calcium in that it is a divalent cation which is partly protein bound (about 45%) and partly ultrafiltrable, and in that it is largely under the control of parathyroid hormone. Hypomagnesaemia stimulates secretion of PTH and hypermagnesaemia inhibits it. PTH secretion leads to release of magnesium from bone, increased renal tubular reabsorption of magnesium and increased absorption from the intestine.

Both hypocalcaemia and hypomagnesaemia increase neuromuscular irritability and hypomagnesaemia is a rare cause of tetany. High concentrations of magnesium depress neuromuscular activity. Rapid elevation of serum magnesium by injection of a magnesium preparation causes magnesium narcosis, which can be reversed by injection of calcium. Magnesium is an activator of the enzyme systems which require thiamine pyrophosphate as a co-factor.

The renal excretion of magnesium is probably at least partly controlled by aldosterone as well as by PHT.

The normal daily diet contains about 12.5 mmol of magnesium mainly in meat, nuts, bananas, citrus fruit, chocolate and green vegetables.

1. Hypomagnesaemia

The causes of hypomagnesaemia are shown in Table 50.

1.1. Causes of hypomagnesaemia

1.1.1. Reduced intake
Magnesium deficiency rarely occurs from deficient intake alone because renal conservation is very efficient. It is found in the Third World in children with protein malnutrition, especially if there is associated diarrhoea. It may occur in patients requiring parenteral nutrition for periods of even less than a week, when the fluids given are magnesium-free.

Table 50. Causes of hypomagnesaemia.

1. Reduced intake
2. Gastrointestinal loss
    2.1. Gastric fluid
    2.2. Fistulae
    2.3. Small bowel resection
    2.4. Diarrhoea
3. Renal loss
    3.1. Recovery from acute renal failure
    3.2. Renal tubular function impairment
    3.3. Diuretics
    3.4. Following major surgery
    3.5. Familial hypokalaemia with hypomagnesaemia
4. Alcoholism
5. Endocrine causes of magnesium loss

1.1.2. Gastrointestinal loss

Magnesium may be lost by prolonged nasogastric suction, loss of fluid from pancreatic and small bowel fistulae, following massive resection of small bowel, and in the chronic diarrhoea and steatorrhoea of other forms of malabsorption. Magnesium is excreted in the faeces as magnesium soaps. A high calcium or low protein diet increases the loss of magnesium.

1.1.3

Renal loss of magnesium occurs in the diuretic phase of acute renal failure but this rarely causes symptoms. It may be due to treatment with thiazide or mercurial diuretics – which may be important for patients also taking digitalis, as digitalis toxicity may be precipitated or made worse by hypomagnesaemia. Excessive urinary loss of magnesium during the first 24 hours after major surgery may lead to transient hypomagnesaemia.

1.1.4. Alcoholism

Depletion of magnesium is often present in alcoholic patients. This is probably due to a combination of factors including a deficient diet with poor absorption and increased urinary loss. Hypomagnesaemia is common after acute withdrawal of alcohol.

1.1.5. Endocrine causes

Hypomagnesaemia may occur in hypoparathyroidism along with hypocalcaemia. It occurs post-operatively in patients with bone disease due to hyperparathyroidism and may be a cause of persistent tetany in spite of a fairly normal serum calcium concentration. It also occurs in primary aldosteronism, diabetic acidosis, hypercalcaemia due to hyperparathyroidism and in hypercalcaemia due to other conditions, and in acute intermittent porphyria with syndrome of inappropriate ADH secretion.

1.2. Symptoms and signs of hypomagnesaemia

The symptoms include tetany, tremor, athetoid movements, irritability and changes in personality, convulsions, increased reflexes, clonus, nystagmus, muscle fasciculations and marked muscle weakness. Tachycardia, hypotension and vasomotor changes with cold, painful peripheries may occur. Anorexia, nausea and vomiting may be present.

1.3. Treatment of hypomagnesaemia

Magnesium sulphate may be given intravenously for treatment of tetany thought to be due to hypomagnesaemia. It may be given as a 1% solution in 5% dextrose (obtained by dilution of 10% or 50% magnesium sulphate), 1 litre being infused over 3–4 hours. Relief of symptoms may not occur for several days, unlike the immediate relief of hypocalcaemic tetany by intravenous injection of calcium. It may also be given intramuscularly, 1–2 g (50% solution) every 2–6 hours, monitoring the level obtained. Intramuscular injection of magnesium sulphate is said to be painful, and I have not given it by this route. If it is to be given by intramuscular injection procaine hydrochloride may be added.

2. Hypermagnesaemia

Hypermagnesaemia is usually due to renal failure. In patients with moderate renal failure hypermagnesaemia may be made worse by giving commercial antacids containing magnesium (Gavison, Gelusil, Aludrox, etc.).

Hypermagnesaemia may be caused by injection of magnesium to control convulsions. It has also followed the use of frequent enemas of magnesium sulphate.

2.1. Symptoms and signs of hypermagnesaemia

These are non-specific and include thirst, sense of heat, nausea, vomiting and a tendency to hypotension due to peripheral vaso-dilatation. Depression of the respiratory centre, coma and finally cardiac arrest occur at very high levels.

2.2. Treatment of hypermagnesaemia

Magnesium-containing drugs should be avoided or used with caution in patients with renal failure. Hydration should be made normal if underhydration is present. Magnesium can be removed by dialysis.

21. Parenteral nutrition

1. Parenteral nutrition

It is generally accepted that parenteral nutrition is an important part of the care of severely injured and critically ill patients. It has also been claimed that full parenteral nutrition improves healing to patients undergoing major surgery and reduces the incidence of complications. There does not seem to be any evidence that a short period of negative nitrogen in previously well-nourished patients increases the complication rate or delays healing. It has been shown that patients undergoing proctocolectomy given 12 g nitrogen daily for about 12 days lose less weight and were in less negative nitrogen balance than patients given glucose only for nutrition, but the complication rate and length of stay in hospital were the same in both groups. In another group of patients undergoing surgery for oesophageal carcinoma, parenteral nutrition reduced the incidence of wound infection only in patients already severely mal-nourished. The loss of a few kilograms body weight is of little importance in normally nourished patients.

The main problem is therefore to identify the patients who require full parenteral nutrition. It was stated recently that in the 600-bed Central Middlesex Hospital just over one per cent of patients were fed enterally or parenterally each year, one quarter of whom were treated parenterally. Severely traumatised patients with multiple injuries, patients who have undergone complicated surgery, especially if sepsis supervenes, patients with extensive burns and those with severe sepsis are all hypercatabolic with high energy requirements. The nitrogen loss in such patients may be about 20–25 g daily, as urea, creatinine and creatine, about 3 times greater than that occurring during starvation and equivalent to about 600–800 g of muscle. Such large losses of nitrogen soon lead to obvious muscle wasting and severe debility. In a patient who is unable to take adequate oral nutritives either voluntarily or by nasogastric tube for 3 days, parenteral feeding should be considered.

Parenteral feeding has many hazards, including mechanical damage by catheters during insertion and afterwards, sepsis, thrombosis occurring in large vessels, and electrolyte imbalance including phosphate depletion. Incompatibilities between solutions and drug additives are common. Severely traumatised patients may develop acute renal failure or liver failure and may have limited capability to utilise infused nutrients. These patients would require treatment in an intensive care unit quite apart from parenteral nutrition, and while the solutions are expensive, relative to the other costs of intensive care the extra cost is not prohibitive and may well be life saving.

Other patients with wasting may and should be identified in ordinary wards. The problem arises as to whether full parenteral nutrition can be carried out there, and as to who will be qualified to carry out the treatment. The use of hypertonic solutions infused into central veins requires the vigilance of an intensive care unit. However, treatment with isotonic solutions (if equally effective) infused into peripheral veins could be carried out in an ordinary ward and reduce the cost.

It has been suggested that in each hospital parenteral nutrition should be the responsibility of a nutrition team. The team would be on-call for parenteral and enteral nutrition, would instruct junior doctors and nursing staff in the procedures and would provide continuity of the service. This plan has obvious advantages, but is not acceptable to everyone as there are many different ideas on correct technique and equipment. Moreover senior doctors often do not like being told how to manage their patients.

2. Planning parenteral nutrition

The provision of calories and nitrogen is calculated on a basis of weight. The daily requirement of calories for ill patients is about 40 kcal/kg (168 J) but may be as high as 50 kcal/kg in hypercatabolic patients. The nitrogen requirement is 0.20–0.30 g/kg/day.

If the plasma protein concentration is already low an infusion of albumen should be given at the begining of therapy.

About 50% of the calories should be given as carbohydrate, the concentration depending on the fluid requirements (calculated in the usual way on replacement of previous day's output and of insensible loss – this volume to include fluids for all purposes). Fat emulsion may provide 30–40% of the daily calorie intake, as fat provides calories without an osmotic load. Protein from amino acid solutions should provide 10–15% of the daily calorie intake.

The nutritional requirements must be tailored to the electrolyte requirements of the individual patients, i.e., the sodium and potassium in the nutrition solutions must be included in the daily requirements. This may be of crucial importance in a patient with acute renal failure or with lesser impairment of renal function. Fat emulsion should not be used as a source of energy in the presence of liver failure.

2.1. Amino acids

Casein hydrolysates were originally used for parenteral feeding but have been superseded (because of side effects) by synthetic amino acid mixtures. These are given as L-isomers because the body cannot utilise D-isomers except for small amounts of D-methionine and D-phenylalanine.

Some amino acid solutions contain added carbohydrate as amino acids alone do not provide energy in readily usable form. However, carbohydrate given with amino acids stimulates insulin secretion and this inhibits the use of body fat as a source of energy. Amino acids have been infused alone to avoid the insulin response and it is claimed that endogenous fat can then be used as a source of calories and the amino acids are then used for tissue repair. This theory has not been confirmed by other studies and it is even claimed that addition of carbohydrate may reduce the amount of amino acid needed to achieve positive nitrogen balance. In any case insulin stimulates protein synthesis. It is, therefore, not clear whether it is better to give amino acids alone or with added carbohydrate.

Solutions available, with their nitrogen and electrolyte content are shown in Table 51. Aminosol is the only one of these solutions containing phosphate but its high sodium content needs to be considered in some patients. Perifusin BDH is isotonic and does not contain carbohydrate but is the most expensive way of giving nitrogen (£17.30/10 g non-glycine).

Table 51. Amino acid solutions.

Solution	Volume	K Calories	Nitrogen g	Sodium mmol	Potassium mmol
Aminosol 10%	1000	320	12.7	160	0.5
Trophysan 10%	1000	564 (sorbitol)	6.7	6	8.0
Vamin 7%	1000	650 (fructose)	9.4	50	20.0
Aminoplex 5	1000	1000 (sorbitol and ethanol)	5.0	35	15
Aminoplex 12	1000	315	12.4	50	30
Perifusin BDH	1000	132	5.0		

2.2. Carbohydrates

Glucose is readily metabolised by all tissues provided insulin is available. However, many severely ill patients have high serum glucose levels with very low insulin concentrations. These patients benefit from regular additional insulin. 1 litre of 5% glucose provides only 200 calories. More concentrated solutions of 20% and 50% can be given but only through catheters inserted into central veins.

Fructose is used in 20% solution and can be substituted for glucose. It has been claimed that insulin is not required for its metabolism, but this is not strictly true. It should not be given to severely debilitated patients or those with hypoxaemia or shock where it may lead to severe lactic acidosis.

Sorbitol is used in 30% solution. It is converted into glucose and fructose. It has no practical advantage over glucose. It is a powerful osmotic diuretic.

Xylitol is a pentose sugar which has been used as an energy source. Acute renal failure has been reported after its use and it has been banned in the USA, UK and Australia. Ethanol is a useful source of energy, 1 g yielding 7.1 calories. The amount infused should not exceed 10 g/hr. Some amino acid solutions contain ethanol and if infused rapidly they may cause confusion, flushing and tachycardia which may be mistaken for septicaemia.

2.3. Fat solutions

Intralipid is a soya bean oil emulsion which provides 9.3.calories/g fat. It is also a valuable source of phosphate as phospholipids.

Fat emulsion should be given some hours before blood samples are to be taken for biochemical estimations, to avoid hyperlipidaemia.

Very recently fat embolization has been described following intravenous administration of fat solutions to very ill patients. It may be unwise to give intravenous fat solutions in these circumstances.

2.4. Minerals

Calcium, phosphate, magnesium and zinc must be given as well as nutrients. A convenient method of ensuring adequate intake of these essential substances is the use of the commercial preparation GluCoplex 1000 (24% glucose) or GluCoplex 1600 (40% glucose). Both contain added phosphate, magnesium and zinc.

3. Method of administration

Peripheral veins can be used for administration of isotonic amino acids and fat emulsions. Even the more concentrated amino acid solutions can be given into peripheral veins for a few days. The concentrated carbohydrate solutions must be given into the subclavian vein. The position of the catheter tip must be checked radiologically to ensure that it is correctly sited.

Strict aseptic technique during insertion of the catheter is essential as sepsis is the greatest hazard of parenteral nutrition. The continuing care of the catheter should be entrusted only to specially trained nurses. The infusion tube should be changed every 24–48 hours.

Septicaemia or infected thrombus are suggested by a spiking temperature chart.

Despite the many problems associated with parenteral nutrition, it has been possible with the use of silastic catheters placed in the right atrium to continue treatment for several years. Some patients have been able to give their own intravenous infusions overnight and live normally by day for long periods.

4. Scheme for parenteral nutrition

4.1. Collection of base-line information

The patient is weighed or weight is estimated. A base-line sample of venous blood is taken for concentrations of urea, electrolytes including bicarbonate, creatinine, calcium, phosphate, magnesium, zinc if available, AST, bilirubin, glucose.

A 24-hour urine collection is commenced for creatinine clearance, protein excretion, urea, creatinine concentration and excretion of electrolytes.

4.2. Preparation for feeding

A catheter is inserted into the subclavian vein and a chest X-ray is taken to check the position of the catheter tip. It is often convenient to maintain a peripheral venous infusion through which drugs may be given, and additional electrolytes given as required, but this dual system can only be used in patients with adequate renal function and maintaining a good urinary output.

4.3

When renal function is normal, excess water and electrolytes can be excreted, but careful recording of fluid intake and output are essential in case urinary volume declines, e.g., if a fall in blood pressure occurs. Daily measurement of sodium and potassium excretion are helpful.

When renal function is not normal, the volume requirements must be based on the volume of the previous day's losses by all routes plus 500 ml for insensible loss (not required if the patient is breathing humidified gases). Sodium and potassium requirements are based on previous day's measured excretion. Underestimation is safer than overestimation.

4.4

A specimen prescription for an adult patient who is not hypercatabolic or in renal failure is given in Table 52. Vitamin requirements may be given as Solivito (Kabivitrium) and Multibionta on alternate days, the latter being given because of increased requirements of B vitamins in glucose metabolism. Vitamin K 10 mg is given intramuscularly once weekly. Patients who are severely mal-nourished or who require prolonged parenteral nutrition should be given trace elements. One ampoule of Addamel given intravenously daily is a convenient way of providing trace elements.

Table 52. Intravenous feeding solutions given as 3 l per 24 hours.

Solution	ml	N g	Kcal	Na mmol	K mmol	Cl mmol	Mg mmol	PO$_4$ mmol	Zn mmol
Aminoplex 12	1000	12.44	312	35	30	67.2	2.5	–	–
GluCoplex 1000	1000	–	1000	50	30	67.0	2.5	18	45.6
GluCoplex 1600	1000	–	1600	50	30	67.0	2.5	18	45.6

Essential fatty acids can be given by a peripheral vein as 500 ml Intralipid twice weekly.

During a period of parenteral feeding the serum urea and electrolytes and glucose concentrations should be estimated daily, plasma proteins, calcium and phosphate concentrations twice weekly. Daily 24-hour urine electrolyte and urea excretions are desirable.

References

1. Johnston IDA: Parenteral nutrition. In: Recent Advances in Surgery. Taylor S (ed.). Edinburgh: Churchill Livingstone, 1977, pp 133–143.
2. Wretlind A: Complete intravenous nutrition. Theoretical and experimental background. Nutr Metabol 14, Suppl: 1–57, 1972.

Further reading

Arruda JAL: Acid-base metabolism. Seminars in Nephrology 1, 3. New York: Grune & Stratton, 1981.

Bahlmann J, Brod J: Disturbances of water and electrolyte balance. Contributions to Nephrology 21. Basel: S. Karger, 1980.

Black DAK: Essentials of fluid balance, 4th ed. Oxford: Blackwell Scientific Publications, 1969.

Brenner BM, Rector FC: The Kidney, Vol 1. Philadelphia: WB Saunders, 1976.

Coe FL: Hypercalcuric states. Seminars in Nephrology 1, 4. New York: Grune & Stratton, 1981.

DeLuca HF: Vitamin D metabolism and function. New York: Springer Verlag, 1979.

Goldberger E: A primer of water, electrolyte and acid-base syndromes, 6th ed. Philadelphia: Lea and Febiger, 1980.

Li AK, Wills MR, Hanson GC: Fluid, electrolytes acid-base and nutrition. London: Academic Press, 1980.

Moore, FD: Fluid and electrolyte management on surgical patients. In: Rhoad's Textbook of Surgery, 5th ed. Hardy JD (ed.). Philadelphia: Lippincott, 1977, pp 20–77.

Pitts RF: Physiology of the kidney and body fluids, 3rd ed. Chicago: Year Book Medical Publishers Incorporated, 1974.

Richet G, Ardaillou R, Amiel C, Paillard M et Kanfer A: Equilibre hydro-électrolytique normal et pathologique, 4th ed. Paris: Ballière, 1979.

Schrier RW: Renal and electrolyte disorders, 2nd ed. Boston: Little Brown & Company, 1980.

Schwartz AB, Lyons H: Acid-base and electrolyte balance. Normal regulation and clinical disorders. New York: Grune & Stratton, 1977.

Zilva JF, Pannall PR: Clinical chemistry in diagnosis and treatment. Aylesbury: Lloyd-Luke, 1979.

Appendix 1

Elements and atomic weights

Name	Symbol	Atomic weight	Valency
Aluminum	Al	26.97	3
Antimony (stibium)	Sb	121.76	3, 5
Arsenic	As	74.91	3, 5
Barium	Ba	137.36	2
Bismuth	Bi	209.00	3, 5
Bromine	Br	79.916	1
Calcium	Ca	40.08	2
Carbon	C	12.01	2, 4
Chlorine	Cl	35.457	1
Chromium	Cr	52.01	2, 3, 6
Cobalt	Co	58.94	2, 3
Copper	Cu	63.57	1, 2
Fluorine	F	19.00	1
Gold (aurum)	Au	197.2	1, 3
Helium (liquid)	He	4.003	0
Hydrogen (liquid)	H	1.008	1
Iodine	I	126.932	1
Iron (ferrum)	Fe	55.85	2, 3
Lead (plumbum)	Pb	207.21	2, 4
Lithium	Li	6.940	1
Magnesium	Mg	24.32	2
Manganese	Mn	54.93	2, 4, 6, 7
Mercury (hydrargyrum)	Hg	200.61	1, 2
Molybdenum	Mo	96.95	3, 4, 6
Nickel	Ni	58.69	2, 3
Nitrogen (liquid)	N	14.008	3, 5
Oxygen (liquid)	O	16.000	2, 3, 4, 8
Palladium	Pd	106.7	2, 4
Phosphorus	P	31.02	3, 5
Platinum	Pt	195.23	2, 4
Potassium (kalium)	K	39.10	1
Radium	Rd or Ra	226.05	2
Radon (niton)	Rn	222.0	0
Selenium	Se	78.96	2, 4, 6

Appendix 1. Continued

Name	Symbol	Atomic weight	Valency
Silicon	Si	28.06	4
Silver (argentum)	Ag	107.880	1
Sodium (natrium)	Na	22.997	1
Strontium	Sr	87.63	2
Sulfur	S	32.06	2, 4, 6
Tin (stannum)	Sn	118.70	2, 4
Tungsten (wolframium)	W	184.0	6
Uranium	U	238.07	4, 6
Vanadium	V	50.95	3, 5
Zinc	Zn	91.22	4

Modified from Appendix 8, Cheigh, Stenzl & Rubin, *Manual of Clinical Nephrology*, The Hague: Martinus Nijhoff, 1981, with kind permission.

Appendix 2

How to make a 24-hour urine collection

1. Decide a suitable time to commence (and end) the test, e.g., 08.00 hours.
2. Empty bladder at exactly 08.00 hours and *discard* the urine (i.e., commence test with an empty bladder).
3. Save *all* urine passed in the bottle provided, *including* the urine passed at exactly 08.00 hours the following morning (i.e., end the test with an empty bladder).

Common sources of error include saving the urine passed at the beginning of the test (which of course belongs to the previous 24 hours); failure to void and save urine before defaecation; failure to save the final specimen; lack of provision of an extra container in case the 24 hour urine collection exceeds 2 litres.

Appendix 3

Guide to assess fluid requirements

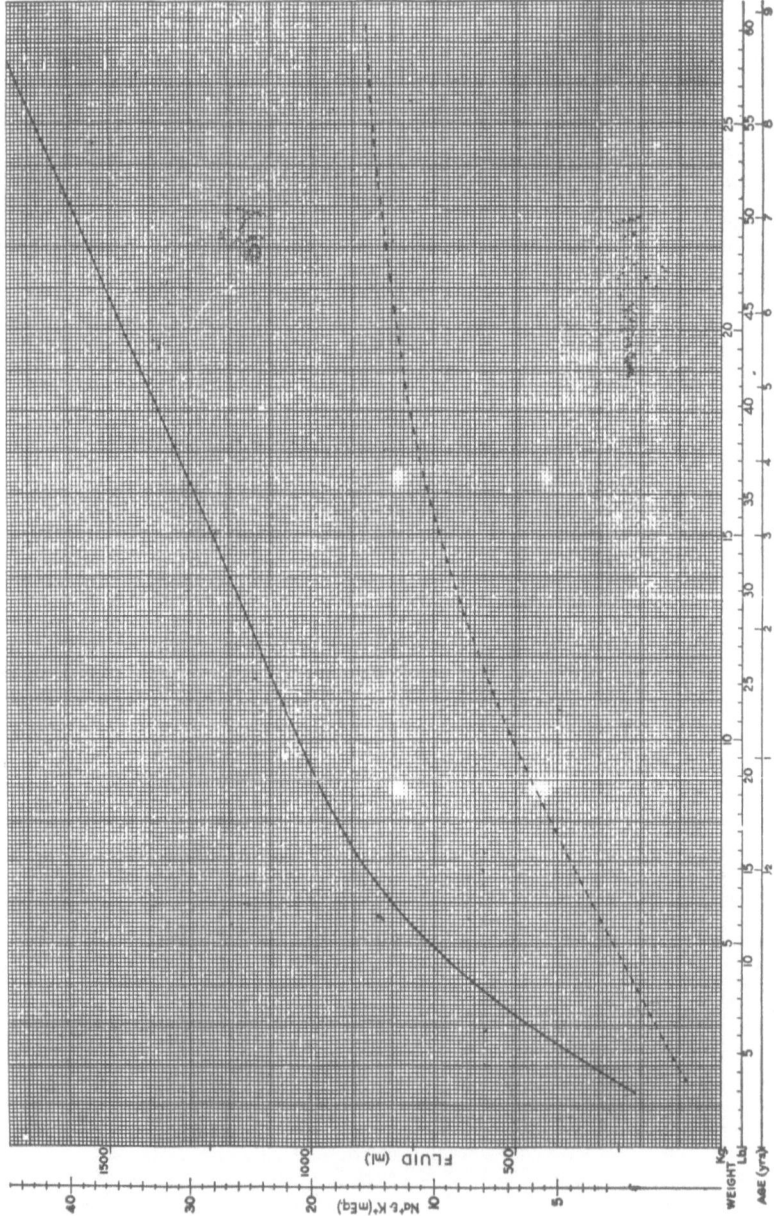

Fig. 1A. chart enabling a rapid assessment of both 24-hour maintenance requirements of Na$^+$, K$^+$ and fluid (solid line), and of 24-hour extra-renal fluid losses under conditions of bed rest in hospital (broken line) in children over 10 days of age. Reproduced by kind permission of Professor I.J. Carré and the Irish Journal of Medical Science (Ir J Med Sc, 135–146, 1965).

Appendix 4

Intravenous administration of drugs

Drugs should be given by continuous infusion only when they must be given very slowly and well diluted (potassium chloride, tetracycline, streptokinase) or when a constant therapeutic effect is required (lignocaine, oxytocin). The necessity for addition of drugs to sterile intravenous fluids can be reduced by the use of ready-prepared dilutions of potassium chloride and lignocaine. A limited range of commercial intravenous fluids containing 20 or 40 millimoles of potassium per litre are available. Some hospital pharmacists produce standard dilutions of lignocaine in dextrose or fructose. Heparin is best given by syringe driven by a constant infusion pump, thus providing more accurate control over dosage, avoiding unnecessary administration of large volumes of infusion fluid, and allowing greater mobility to the patient.

The following *must* be given by continuous infusion:

  Potassium chloride
  Tetracycline
  Amphotericin B
  Streptokinase
  Lignocaine
  Oxytocin
  Flagyl

Intermittent intravenous administration of drugs is preferable to continuous infusion where the attainment of high blood levels is necessary (e.g., most antibiotics). Many antibiotics, such as gentamicin, ampicillin, never reach effective levels when given by continuous infusion either because of rapid clearance from the blood or because of rapid loss of activity in the infusion fluid. Compound vitamin injections (Parentrovite) although often given by constant infusion, can be given by intermittent injection.

Appendix 5

Electrolyte content of antibiotics

Antibiotic		Total electrolyte concentration mmol per g antibiotic	
Approved name	Proprietary name	Oral formulation	Injectable formulation
Amikacin	Amikin	---	–
Amoxycillin	Amoxil	–	2.6 Na$^+$
	Augmentin[a]	1.8 K$^+$	---
Ampicillin	Amfipen	–	---
	Ampiclox[a]	---	1.2 Na$^+$
	Magnapen	0.5 Na$^+$	1.2 Na$^+$
	Penbritin	–	2.7 Na$^+$
	Pentrexyl	–	---
	Vidopen	–	---
Benethamine penicillin	Triplopen[a]	---	0.8 Na$^+$
Benzathine penicillin	Penidural	–	---
	Penidural[a] All-purpose	---	0.5 K$^+$
	Penidural Long-acting	---	–
Benzylpenicillin potassium	Crystapen G	2.7 K$^+$	---
	Penidural[a] All-purpose	---	0.5 K$^+$
Benzylpenicillin sodium	Bicillin	---	1.7 Na$^+$
	Crystamycin[a]	---	0.8 Na$^+$
	Crystapen	---	2.8 Na$^+$
	Triplopen[a]	---	0.8 Na$^+$
Carbenicillin	Pyopen	---	4.7 Na$^+$
Carfecillin	Uticillin	2.1 Na$^+$	---
Cefaclor	Distaclor	–	---
Cefoxitin	Mefoxin	---	2.2 Na$^+$
Cefuroxime	Zinacef	---	2.1 Na$^+$
Cephadrine	Velosef	–	6.0 Na$^+$
Cephalexin	Ceporax	–	---
	Keflex	–	---
Cephaloridine	Ceporin	---	–
Cephalothin	Keflin	---	2.4 Na$^+$
Cephazolin	Kefzol	---	2.1 Na$^+$

Appendix 5. Continued

Antibiotic		Total electrolyte concentration mmol per g antibiotic	
Approved name	Proprietary name	Oral formulation	Injectable formulation
Chloramphenicol	Chloromycetin	–	2.2 Na$^+$
	Kemicetine	---	2.2 Na$^+$
Chlortetracycline	Aureomycin	–	---
	Deteclo^a	–	---
Clavulanic acid	Augmentin^a	0.63 K$^+$	---
Clindamycin	Dalacin C	–	–
Clomocycline	Megaclor	1.88 Na$^+$ (capsule) 0.95 Ca^{++} (liquid)	---
Cloxacillin	Ampiclox^a	---	1.2 Na$^+$
	Orbenin	2.1 Na$^+$	2.1 Na$^+$
Colistin	Colomycin	–	–
Co-trimoxazole	Bactrim	–	–
	Septrim	–	–
Demeclocycline	Deteclo^a	–	---
	Ledermycin	–	---
Doxycycline	Vibramycin	–	---
Erythromycin	Erythrocin	–	–
	Erythromid	–	---
	Erythroped	–	---
	Ilisone	–	---
	Ilotycin	–	---
	Retcin	–	---
Flucloxacillin	Floxapen	2.0 Na$^+$	2.0 Na$^+$
Fusidate salt	Fucidin	1.9 Na$^+$	0.4 Na$^+$
Gentamicin	Cidomycin	---	0.03 Na$^+$
	Genticin	---	0.02 Na$^+$
Kanamycin	Kannasyn	---	0.26 Na$^+$
	Kantrex	–	0.33 Na$^+$
Linomycin	Lincocin	–	–
Lymecycline	Tetralysal	–	---
Methacycline	Rondomycin	– (capsule) 2.1 Ca^{++} (liquid)	---
Methicillin	Celbenin	---	2.4 Na$^+$
Neomycin	Mycifradin	---	–
	Nivemycin	–	---
Novobiocin	Albamycin	1.6 Na$^+$	1.6 Na$^+$
Oxytetracycline	Berkmycen	– (tablet)	---
	Imperacin	1.0 Ca^{++} (syrup)	
	Terramycin	– (tablet) 1.0 Ca^{++} (syrup)	---
Phenethicillin	Broxil	2.5 K$^+$	---
Phenoxymethyl penicillin	V-cil-K	2.6 K$^+$	---
Pivmecillinam	Selexid	–	–

194

Appendix 5. Continued

Antibiotic		Total electrolyte concentration mmol per g antibiotic	
Approved name	Proprietary name	Oral formulation	Injectable formulation
Polymyxin B	Aerosporin	---	–
Procaine penicillin	Various brands	---	–
Spectinomycin	Trobicin	---	–
Spiramycin	Rovamycin	---	–
Streptomycin	---	---	–
Talampicillin	Talpen	–	---
Tetracycline	Achromycin (various brands)	–	– (IV) 2.5 Mg^{++} (IM)
Tobramycin	Nebcin	---	–

[a] Composite antibiotic: concentration per unit, e.g., tablet, capsule, vial
--- = Antibiotic not available in this formulation
– = No electrolyte present in this formulation

Appendix 6

Drugs which cause proteinuria and nephrotic syndrome

Drug	Use	Nephrotic syndrome	Other known renal effects	Contributing factor	Recovery of renal function
Aloes	purgative	+	acute renal failure via K$^+$ loss		±
Amphotericin B	antifungal antibiotic	–	acute renal failure		±
Bacitracin	antibiotic	–	tubular dysfunction		+
Bismuth salts	antacid	+	acute renal failure		+
Cephaloridine	antibiotic	–	–	high doses	+
Dapsone	antileprotic dermatitis herpetiformis	+	haematuria	deficiency of G6PD	+
Diloxanide	amoebiasis	–	–	–	+
Disodium edetate	chelating agent	–	–	–	+
Ethosuximide	anticonvulsant	–	–	–	+
Gold salts	antirheumatoid	+	–	–	±
Halothane	anaesthetic	+	–	–	+
Ipecacuanha	emetic, expectorant	–	–	–	+
Male fern	anthelmintic	–	–	impaired renal function	+
Mercury	skin-lightening cream	–	–	–	–
Mersalyl and other mercurials	diuretic	+	–	–	±
Methsuximide	anticonvulsant	+	–	–	+
Naproxen	antirheumatoid	–	–	–	+?
Paramethadione	anticonvulsant	+	–	–	+
Penicillin	antibiotic	–	–	–	+
Penicillamine	antirheumatoid Wilson's disease cystinuria	+	–	–	±
Pheneturide	anticonvulsant	+	–	–	+
Phenindione	anticoagulant	+	–	acute renal failure	+
Phenolphthalein	laxative	–	–	–	+
Phensuximide	anticonvulsant	–	–	–	+

Drug	Use	Nephrotic syndrome	Other known renal effects	Contributing factor	Recovery of renal function
Phenylbutazone	antirheumatoid	−	−	−	±
Polymyxins	antibiotics	−	tubular dysfunction	−	+
Probenecid	uricosuric	+	tubular dysfunction	−	?
Sodium aminosalicylate	antitubercular agent	−	acute renal failure	−	+
Sodium cacodylate	antisyphilitic	−	−	−	±
Sodium calcium edetate	chelating agent	−	−	−	+
Suramin	trypanocide	−	acute renal failure	−	+
Theophylline monoethanol-amine	bronchodilator	−	−	−	+
Tolbutamide	hypoglycaemic agent	+	−	−	+
Troxidone	anticonvulsant	+	−	−	+

Reproduced by courtesy of Oxford University Press from 'Iatrogenic Diseases', D'Arcy PF, Griffin JP (eds.) 2nd ed. 1979, McGeown MG, p. 267.

Index